BEST
OF
TRADITIONAL CHINESE
MEDICINE

XIE ZHU-FAN, M.D.

NEW WORLD PRESS, BEIJING, CHINA

First Edition 1995

Copyright by **New World Press**, Beijing, China. All rights reserved. No part of this book may be reproduced in any form or by any means without permission in writing from the publisher.

ISBN 7-80005-228-1

Published by
NEW WORLD PRESS
24 Baiwanzhuang Road, Beijing 100037, China
Distributed by
CHINA INTERNATIONAL BOOK TRADING CORPORATION
35 Chengongzhuang Xilu, Beijing 100044, China
P.O. Box 399, Beijing, China

Printed in the People's Republic of China

CONTENTS

FOREWORD	1
CHAPTER I INTRODUCTION TO BASIC MEDICAL THEORIES	9
Theory of *Yin-Yang* — Law of Unity of Opposites	9
Concept of Wholism	11
The Human Body	12
Cause of Disease	16
Differentiation of Syndromes	21
Principles of Prevention and Treatment	23
CHAPTER II IMMUNITY IN TRADITIONAL CHINESE MEDICINE	25
Brief Historical Review	25
Theoretical Aspect of Immunity in Traditional Chinese Medicine	26
Medicinal Herbs and Immunity	29
Examples of Herbal Treatment in Diseases Related to Immune Disorders	37
CHAPTER III HERBS VS. INFECTIONS	42
Differentiation of Syndromes in Acute Infections	43
Herbal Therapies of Acute Infections	45
Pharmacological Studies of the Herbal Therapies	48
Traditional Treatment of Chronic Infections	54
Examples of Herbal Treatment for Infectious Diseases	54
CHAPTER IV USE OF TONICS IN TRADITIONAL CHINESE MEDICINE	61
Deficiency Syndromes	61
Classification of Tonics	63
Modern Research on Tonics	66

Tonic Treatment for Common Diseases	71
CHAPTER V TRADITIONAL CHINESE MEDICINE AND THE AGING	82
Basic Features of Aging	82
Cause of Senility	83
Approaches to Prevent Senility and Retard Aging	84
CHAPTER VI TRADITIONAL CHINESE MEDICINE IN THE TREATMENT OF CANCER	93
Traditional Concept of Cancer	93
Herbal Medication of Cancer	95
Herbal Medicines in the Prevention of Cancer	103
CHAPTER VII ACUPUNCTURE AND MOXIBUSTION	106
Meridians and Acupuncture Points	106
Technique and Methods	108
Indications and Contraindications	110
Examples of Acupuncture Treatment of Common Diseases	111
Therapeutic Mechanism	117
Acupuncture to Combat Pain	121
CHAPTER VIII QI (VITAL ENERGY) AND QIGONG	125
Concept of *Qi*	125
General Methods of *Qigong*	126
Physiological Changes During *Qigong*	130
Treatment of Hypertension with *Qigong*	131
Treatment of Other Diseases with *Qigong*	133
Qigong Deviations	134
About "Out-going *Qi*" ("External *Qi*")	134
CHAPTER IX DIETOTHERAPY IN TRADITIONAL CHINESE MEDICINE	139
The Five Tastes — Pungent, Sweet, Sour, Bitter and Salty	140
The Four Properties — Hot, Warm, Cool and Cold	141
Diet to Combat Pathogenic Factors	143
Diet for Strengthening Body Resistance	145
Food Taboos	148
INDEX	151

FOREWORD

Traditional Chinese medicine has a long history, which can be traced back at least 2,000 or 3,000 years. Records of various diseases, such as dental caries and parasitoses, have been found in inscriptions on tortoise shells and bones excavated in the 13th century B.C. ruins near Anyang, Henan Province. In the *Shi Jing* (*Book of Poems*), a collection of verses compiled in the 12th century B.C., a number of herbs, such as fritillary, motherwort, asiatic plantain, and others, are mentioned.

According to *Shi Ji* (*Records of the Historian*) written in 104-91 B.C., the celebrated physician Bian Que, who lived in the 5th century B.C., successfully employed diagnostic pulse feeling and acupuncture treatment to rescue the crown prince of the State of Guo who was in shock and proclaimed by the court to have just expired. The technique of pulse feeling and acupuncture was thus developed as early as the 5th century B.C.

Medical writings dating back to the 3rd and as early as the 8th century B.C. were found among the books made of silk discovered in Tomb No. 3 excavated in 1973 near Mawangdui Village in Changsha, Hunan Province. They include *Mai Fa* (*Methods of Pulse Feeling*), *Zu Bi Shi Yi Mai Jiu Jing* (*Eleven Meridians for Moxibustion of the Arms and Feet*), *Wu Shi Er Bing Fang* (*Prescriptions for Fifty-two Diseases*), and others.

Around the 3rd century B.C., under the influence of the prevailing materialistic outlook and simple dialectics, particularly the philosophical concepts of *Yin-Yang* and the Five Elements, practical experience accumulated in the previous centuries was summed up into a unique system of medical theories. *Huang Di Nei Jing* (*The Yellow Emperor's Canon of Medicine*), also known simply as *Nei Jing* (*Canon of Medicine*), is the earliest and most comprehensive medical classic from both theoretical and clinical point of view. It covers a variety of subjects, including man and nature, human anatomy and physiology, causes of disease, pathology, diagnosis, differentiation of symptoms and signs, treatment, disease prevention, health preservation, and so forth. The theories of *Yin-*

Yang, visceral organs and meridians have since become the foundation of traditional Chinese medicine.

Around the 2nd century B.C., *Shen Nong Ben Cao Jing* (*The Divine Peasant's Herbal* or simply *The Herbal*) appeared as China's earliest pharmacological work, in which 365 kinds of drugs were divided, according to their toxicity, into three categories: superior, common and inferior.

Clinical medicine continued to develop, both in terms of theory and in making discoveries of effective herbs. At about the beginning of the 3rd century A.D., Zhang Zhongjing wrote *Treatise on Febrile and Miscellaneous Diseases*, a book on diagnosis and treatment of fevers and other miscellaneous diseases. The *Treatise* classifies fevers into six groups based on the meridians; classifies other diseases according to the pathological changes of visceral organs; and outlines a system of diagnosis and treatment of diseases based on analysis and differentiation of syndromes with tested prescriptions. It was a work which laid the foundation for clinical practice in traditional Chinese medicine. Later divided into two books, *Shang Han Lun* (*Treatise on Febrile Diseases*) and *Jin Kui Yao Lue Fang Lun* (*Synopsis of Prescriptions of the Golden Chamber*), the *Treatise*, in combination with *Canon of Medicine* and *The Herbal*, have become the most influential works in the field.

At about the same period of Zhang Zhongjing, a famous surgeon called Hua Tuo performed laparotomy under drug anesthesia. This is described in *Hou Han Shu* (*History of the Later Han Dynasty*) as follows: When a disease affected a visceral organ and neither herbal medication nor acupuncture proved effective, Hua Tuo gave the patient a dose of herbs *mafeisan* (an anesthetic probably containing datura flower as its principal ingredient) in wine, rendering the patient unconscious. Hua Tuo then opened the patient's abdominal cavity and removed the "accumulated mass."

Also in the 3rd century A.D., *Zhen Jiu Jia Yi Jing* (*A Classic of Acupuncture and Moxibustion*) was compiled. This work gave comprehensive information on the location and therapeutic effects of the "points" and detailed the experiences gained in these treatments.

A monograph of pulse diagnosis entitled *Mai Jing* (*Classic on the Pulse*) was compiled at that time, in which 24 different patterns and their diagnostic significance were described in detail. This book and *Classic of Acupuncture and Moxibustion* were taken to Japan in the 7th century; both were later listed among the textbooks by the Japanese government for a medical decree. Pulse feeling, introduced also to the Arabs, influenced Arabian medicine as reflected in the voluminous work *Canon* by the celebrated physician Avicenna.

From the 4th to the 18th century there was steady development in the various fields of traditional medicine. Different schools introduced new points of view and diversified herbal recipes, therapeutics prospered.

Clinical medicine, consequently, became more and more specialized. In the 13th century, 13 medical specialities were established, including internal medicine, pediatrics, gynecology and obstetrics, ophthalmology, stomatology and dentistry, pharyngo-laryngology, bone-setting, traumatology, acupuncture and moxibustion. Apart from herbal medicines, acupuncture and moxibustion, other forms of treatment were developed: couching of cataracts with needles (5th century); creating false teeth with amalgam (7th century); treatment of vertebra fracture by suspension, reduction and other means (12th century).

In the middle of the 17th century, epidemics arose outside the range of previous medical experience. A school of thought in the field of febrile disease forwarded the theory that respiratory and digestive infections were the cause of these epidemics. From the 18th century to the early 19th century, books on epidemic febrile disease began to catalogue experiences of diagnosing and treating these diseases. Some of the treatments, such as those for diphtheria, epidemic encephalitis, and others, have been proven effective today.

Of the various breakthroughs in traditional Chinese medicine, one worth mentioning is the use of variolation or inoculation to prevent smallpox. By the 16th century, variolation was widely used in China, and in the 17th century, Russia sent doctors to China to learn the method. It was only after vaccination was initiated by Jenner in 1796 that variolation was abandoned.

As for Chinese materia medica, the number of medicinal substances and prescriptions continued to grow. In the 6th century, when *Shen Nong's Herbal* had fallen behind clinical needs, a new materia medica titled *Ben Cao Jing Ji Zhu* (*Commentaries on Materia Medica*) was produced, in which 730 medicines were classified according to their sources and therapeutic applications. In 1659 *Xin Xiu Ben Cao (Revised Materia Medica)* was compiled, listing 844 medicinal substances. This pharmacopoeia sponsored by the imperial court was the first officially issued in China, as well as the first to come out in the world.

In 1478, the celebrated physician and naturalist Li Shizhen compiled *Ben Cao Gang Mu* (*Compendium of Materia Medica*), a 52-volume encyclopedia of 1,892 medicines with illustrations and 11,000 prescriptions. Having been translated in whole or part into Japanese, English, German, French, Latin and Russian, it has become a masterpiece known the world over. When Charles Darwin quoted from what he called "the ancient Chinese encyclopedia," he was referring to this great work. Traditional Chinese medicine has thus both contributed to the health of the Chinese people and influenced the development of medical science in many other countries as well.

For various historical reasons, however, traditional Chinese medicine developed more slowly than Western medicine in the 19th century and the first half of the 20th century. There was even a trend in China for several decades to eliminate the traditional medical system and replace it with modern Western medicine.

Despite these changes, most Chinese people continued to believe in traditional medicine. In the first place, it has been proven to work even with diseases that can't be cured by modern medicine. Secondly, medicinal herbs have few side effects. Thirdly, though unable to be explained by modern medicine, it has guided clinical practice effectively. This point in particular is interesting to unprejudiced medical professionals.

The situation in China since the middle of this century has radically changed. Great advances have been made, particularly in terms of research. Today a combination of traditional and modern scientific methods is applied; new levels have been reached in both basic theory and clinical applications.

Experimental research and laboratory studies have revealed some of the mysteries of traditional Chinese medical theory. For example, the notion of "kidney" in Chinese medicine is not just the organ that excretes urine; it is a larger functional system that stores the essence of life which controls reproduction, growth and development and is closely related to the brain, marrow and bones. Though some may dispute this hypothesis, it is a fact that many diseases such as sterility, sexual impotence, aplastic anemia, lumbago and impaired memory in the aged are due to deficiency of the kidney. Most cases can be relieved to some extent with herbal medicines to reinforce the kidney. Recent studies have revealed that when the kidney is in a weakened state, hypofunction of the hypothalamic-pituitary-adrenocortical and gonadal system occurs; therapy to reinforce the kidney can readjust the function of the endocrine system. The concept of "kidney" in traditional Chinese medicine therefore actually refers, besides the urinary system, to the endocrine system, particularly the pituitary-adrenocortical-gonadal system.

The wonderful results of acupuncture as a medical treatment have already been widely recognized. Without elucidation of the therapeutic mechanisms involved, however, it could not be taken as a well-grounded branch of medical science. Recent studies have revealed what happen during acupuncture treatment: the effect on the autonomic nervous function, improvement of local blood circulation, and enhancement of cellular immunity. Inhibition of the nervous system and increase of endorphin (a morphine-like substance produced in the nervous system that acts as a pain killer) in the brain during acupuncture is a more acceptable explanation than the vague hypothesis about removal of obstruction to the *qi* (vital energy) and blood flow along the meridians.

Medicines in Chinese pharmacology are classified into four main categories according to their basic properties: "cold," "hot," "warm" and "cool." Syndromes, as well, are so classified, heat and cold being the basic properties. Traditionally, these concepts have been explained by *yin* and *yang*: cold syndromes are caused by decline of *yang*, and heat syndromes by exuberance of *yang*; hot drugs promote *yang*, cold drugs suppress *yang*. Research into the matter has revealed that cold syndromes are characterized by diminished sympathetic function and/or increased parasympathetic function as well as changes in corresponding transmitters at various levels. Herbal medicines used to treat cold and heat syndromes produce the opposite effect on the autonomic nervous system and transmitters. The traditional delineation of cold and heat syndromes thus refers in part to autonomic processes, including reactivity of tissues and cells to their corresponding transmitters. And classification of medicinal herbs into cold-natured and hot-natured drugs is related to their actions on autonomic nervous processes and the reactivity of tissues and cells to their corresponding transmitters. Such classification speaks of basic pharmacological actions which may be somewhat neglected in modern medicine.

In terms of clinical study, more and more extensive research has been conducted. Often traditional differentiation of syndromes is combined with modern diagnosis, and Western medical criteria for assessing therapeutic effects are employed. Much of the research is actually a reevaluation of traditional treatment from a modern perspective.

Traditional Chinese medicine often produces satisfactory results, even with diseases Western medicine hasn't yet found the answer for, such as epidemic hemorrhagic fever, chronic viral hepatitis, chronic atrophic gastritis, abnormal fetal position, retinal vein obstruction, scleroderma, and thromboangiitis obliterans. The need for surgery has been thwarted in some cases, and in the field of orthopedics, fractures have been treated successfully with traditional therapeutic methods. For example, instead of extensive fixation and complete rest, a proper combination of motion and immobilization is recommended, in which only the fractured part is fixed, and the joints and soft tissues surrounding allowed to move. Such treatment has been proven to accelerate the healing time by one-third and shorten the course of treatment by one half.

Study of medicinal herbs is another important field of research which has developed traditional therapies and recipes to new usage and indications. The most striking achievements have been made in therapies for blood-activating and stasis-removing. So-called "blood stasis" in traditional Chinese medicine refers to a variety of conditions including blood congestion, extravasation, thrombosis and any other pathological factor that leads to retarded or impeded blood flow. Medicinal herb recipes used in this therapy work to inhibit blood platelet aggregation, promote fibrolysis, inhibit thrombosis, improve microcirculation, accelerate the absorption of extravasated blood, and modulate the immune function. The therapy has been used successfully in cases of keloids, ischemic cerebrovascular disease, chronic glomerulonephritis, collagen diseases, and in the prevention of ABO neonatal hemolytic disease.

Successful treatments that have integrated Western and traditional Chinese medicine are worth mentioning specially. Because of their different view-points, each aims at different aspect or link in the pathogenetic chain. For instance, in the treatment of a bacteria infection, Western medicine uses antibiotics to destroy the bacteria while traditional medical treatment aims to enhance the patient's immunity. In a simple case, where appropriate antibiotics are available, the antibacterial agent alone will suffice; but in a complicated case where the disease becomes protracted in spite of the antibiotics, a supplement of traditional Chinese medicine yields satisfactory results.

Another approach to the integration of these systems is the use of medicinal herbs or other traditional therapies to minimize the side effects of Western drugs. This is particularly valuable in cases of corticosteroid therapy, chemotherapy and radiotherapy.

In conclusion, over the past 40 years, traditional medicine in China has come a long way. Not only have many historical achievements been confirmed by modern science, but considerable development has also been made. This branch of medicine is sure to make more contributions to the future health of humankind.

In preparing this book, the author concentrated primarily on the exposition of general medical theories and principles of treatment. Clinical approaches and illustrations are also provided. The data cited were obtained in controlled studies under scientific conditions. The title, therefore, ''Best of Traditional Chinese Medicine'' means not only excellent, but also the best researched.

Though some terms in traditional Chinese medicine are the same as those in Western medicine, they may mean quite different things. There is, for example, a marked distinction in the conception of the structure and functions of the visceral organs: the heart, liver, spleen, lung, and kidney. These terms are italicized (throughout the book) to remind readers to think of them in their traditional sense and avoid confusing them with the notions of Western medicine.

CHAPTER I

INTRODUCTION TO BASIC MEDICAL THEORIES

Owing to their different historical backgrounds, there are striking differences between traditional Chinese medicine and Western medicine, not only in practice, but particularly in terms of theory. Traditional Chinese medical theories were formulated by summing up practical experience in the light of ancient Chinese philosophy. These theories, though established thousands of years ago, are still widely adopted by contemporary traditional medical doctors.

Theory of *Yin-Yang*
— Law of Unity of Opposites

Yin and *yang* are two topographic terms used to designate the shady and the sunny sides of a hill. Just as anything under the sun has two sides: the sunny side and the shady side (even when the sun is directly above, the bottom will be shady), *yin* and *yang* represent the two sides of an object or phenomenon. The theory of *yin-yang* in ancient Chinese philosophy was used to epitomize and explain the law of change in nature. According to this theory, everything in the universe has two opposite aspects: *yin* and *yang*, which are in conflict and at the same time interdependent; any change is attributed to the *yin-yang* change within it. This is the law of the unity of opposites. With respect to medicine, the following points can be summarized:

I. Opposition and Interdependence of *Yin* and *Yang*

The words *yin* and *yang* can be used either as attributive adjectives or as nouns. As attributive adjectives, they represent the basic properties of two opposites. In this sense, they mean not only shady and sunny, but refer to a wider range of opposite properties: cold and hot, slow and rapid, dark and bright, heavy and light, quiescent and moving, inhibited and excited, masculine and feminine, lower and upper, interior and exterior, and so on. For example, the meridians running through the medial aspect of the limbs are called *yin* meridians, while those running through the lateral aspect are called *yang* meridians. Light yellow discoloration of the skin and sclera in chronic progress without fever is called *yin*-jaundice; bright yellow discoloration of the skin and sclera with acute onset and fever is called *yang*-jaundice. The *yin-yang* philosophical concept of opposition predominates in traditional Chinese medicine.

Yin and *yang* are also used as nouns. In this sense, they usually represent the most important pair of opposites in the human body, i.e., the substantial and the functional. Therefore, a deficiency of *yin* means the body is lacking structural materials or nutritional substances, while insufficiency of *yang* refers to a decrease in function or metabolism.

Although *yin* and *yang* are in opposition to each other, they are mutually dependent. Neither can exist in isolation. Without "upper," there would be no "lower"; without "exterior," there would be no "interior;" without "moving," there would be no "quiescent." All opposites exist as such, just as the head and tail of a coin.

The most illustrative example of *yin-yang* interdependence is the interrelationship between substance and function. Only with ample substance can the human body function in a healthy way; and only when the functional processes are in good condition, can the essential substances be appropriately replenished.

II. Waxing-Waning and Transformation of *Yin* and *Yang*

The opposites in all objects and phenomena are in constant motion and change: The gain, growth and advance of the one mean the loss, decline and retreat of the other. However, such waxing and waning of *yin-yang* must proceed within certain limits to maintain a dynamic balance for normal development. This concept was derived from meteorological phenomena, particularly seasonal changes in the year. As heat is represented by *yang*, and coolness by *yin*, in spring *yang* gradually increases while *yin* declines, so that the days become warmer and warmer. When this waxing-waning reaches a certain level, summer comes. After the hottest days in mid-summer, waxing of *yang* and waning of *yin* turn to waxing of *yin* and waning of *yang*, and autumn ensues. It is such the weather transforms, through alternation of opposites, from cold to hot, and from hot to cold. Because natural phenomena are balanced in the constant flux of alternating *yin* and *yang* (such as the alternation of day and night, and the waxing and waning of the moon), the change and transformation of *yin-yang* has been taken as a universal law.

In light of this philosophical concept, traditional Chinese medicine holds that human life is a physiological process in constant motion and change. For instance, the functional processes (*yang*) consuming a certain amount of nutritional substances (*yin*) represent the waning of *yin* and waxing of *yang*. The formation and storing of nutritional substances that consume functional energy represent the waxing of *yin* and waning of *yang*.

Under normal conditions, the waxing and waning of *yin* and *yang* are kept within certain bounds, reflecting a dynamic equilibrium of the physiological processes. When the balance is lost, disease occurs. There are four typical cases of imbalance which may result in disease: excess of *yin*, excess of *yang*, deficiency of *yin*, and deficiency of *yang*. The clinical features of each are discussed later in this chapter.

Concept of Wholism

One of the distinguishing features of traditional Chinese medicine is that the human body is viewed as an organic whole. Although the body is composed of various organs and tissues, all are always connected to each other. The connective system includes meridians (also called channels) and collaterals. Meridians and collaterals are the lines along which blood, vital energy and the impetus to functional processes move. Meridians are the cardinal lines, and collaterals are the branches at various levels, which form a structural network.

There has been much dispute in China and abroad about the morphological or histological structure of meridians and collaterals. According to modern research, this system refers chiefly to the nerves, blood vessels, and probably lymphatic vessels. This issue is discussed further in Chapter VII.

Wholism also refers to the unity of the human body and the natural world. On the one hand, the natural world constantly influences the body, and on the other hand, the body adapts to conform to variations in the natural environment.

The concept of wholism is based on the ancient philosophy of the five elements. As with *yin-yang*, the doctrine of five elements— wood, fire, earth, metal and water— was an ancient philosophical concept used to explain the composition of and phenomena in the physical universe. It stresses different properties of the elements and their interrelationships; though the world is in confusion, things and events are related to each other. Later introduced into traditional Chinese medicine, the concept expounds the unity of the human body and the natural world, and the physiological and pathological relationships between various organs and tissues.

A body needs both food and air from the natural world, and lives under constant influence of the weather. Food, by analogy, has properties similar to the five elements. It can be divided into five tastes: sour, bitter, sweet, pungent, and salty, each with its own nutritional value. The weather, as well, can be likened to the five elements. For example, winter is analogous with water, and summer analogous with fire. Variations of food and changes of weather influence the body, which in return should respond properly so that the body can adapt to the external environment. The visceral organs, as well as other organs and tissues, have similar properties to the five elements; they interact physiologically and pathologically as the five elements do. The relationships between the five elements can be classified as such: mutually promoting and restraining under physiological conditions; and encroaching and violating under pathological conditions. By mutually promoting and restraining, functions of the various systems are coordinated and homeostasis maintained. By encroaching and violating, pathological changes can be explained and complications predicted.

The Human Body

Influenced by dialectics and a retarded development of the natural sciences, traditional Chinese medicine is quite different from Western medicine with regard to the structure and function of the human body. The core lies in the visceral organs, which are referred to rather as comprehensive systems of physiological function than as anatomical entities. Among them, the *heart*, *liver*, *spleen*, *lung* and *kidney* are the most important systems; all other organs and tissues are viewed in connection with them.

Traditionally, the *heart* is seen as "ruler of all organs" in charge of blood circulation and mental activity. The word *heart* in traditional Chinese medicine refers to both the cardiovascular system and the higher nervous system.

The *liver* is "a viscus of temperament" in charge of emotional activity. It works to store blood, secrete bile, and control the muscles. The word *liver* refers not only to the liver itself, but also to certain parts of the central nervous system and autonomous nervous system.

The *spleen* functions to transform and transport nutrients and water, nourishing the muscles and limbs and determining the body's constitution. Normal functioning protects the body against pathogens. The word *spleen* refers both to the digestive system and the immune system as well as the functional system in charge of energy and water metabolism.

The *lung*, aside from respiration, controls the vital energy and superficial body resistance and regulates the circulation of body fluid. The word *lung* means the whole respiratory system and part of the immune system; it is also related to water metabolism.

The *kidney* is much more than the organ that secretes urine. It stores the essence of life, either inborn or acquired, and is in charge of reproduction, growth and development. The brain, marrow and bones are all related to the *kidney*. In addition, it helps the *lung* inhale air. Modern research has revealed that the *kidney* actually refers to the urogenital system, endocrine system (particularly the pituitary-adrenal and pituitary-gonadal axes), a part of the immune system and higher nervous system.

The concept of the five visceral organs is quite different from that in Western medicine. It refers to five or more functional systems rather than anatomical entities. In order to avoid confusion, when used in the traditional sense, these terms are printed in italics. The following substitutions, though not very precise, may also be used in most cases:

Liver can be read as the system that controls emotional activities, muscle action, bile secretion and blood storage.

Heart can be read as "heart" and/or "higher nervous system," according to the context.

Spleen can be read as the system responsible for digestion, absorption, assimilation and energy metabolism.

Lung can be read as "respiratory system."

Kidney can be read as the system which works to secrete urine and provide vital essence for heredity, reproduction, development, as well as replenishing the brain, nourishing the bones and producing marrow.

So far as immune functions are concerned, all the above may be involved, but particularly the *lung*, *spleen* and *kidney*.

Apart from the visceral organs, other organs and tissues make up the body: the stomach, small and large intestines, gallbladder, urinary bladder, brain, sensory organs, bones, muscle, blood vessels, and so forth. Since the traditional concepts of these organs and tissues differ little from the modern concepts, no more discussion will be presented in this chapter. The only point to be stressed is that the five visceral organs: the *liver*, *heart*, *spleen*, *lung* and *kidney* are the core of structure and function; and all the other organs and tissues should be viewed in connection with them. The bladder, for example, is closely related to the *kidney*. Some urinary bladder disturbances are attributed to dysfunction of the *kidney* and treated in those terms. And as the *lung* is closely related with the large intestine, purgation of the large intestine with cathartics may help treat *lung* infections. Generally speaking, the relationships between the five visceral organs and other organs and tissues are as follows:

Liver is closely related to the gallbladder, tendons, and eyes. *Heart* is related to the small intestine, blood vessels, and tongue. *Spleen* is related to the stomach, muscles, flesh, and mouth. *Lung* is related to the large intestine, body surface, and nose. *Kidney* is related to the urinary bladder, bones, and ears.

The visceral organs and other organs and tissues need *qi*, blood, vital essence, body fluid and nutrients to carry out their functional processes.

1. *Qi*

This concept, formulated in ancient times, describes *qi* as the basic particles which constitute the cosmos and produce everything in the world through their movements and changes. In traditional medicine, *qi* in its physiological sense refers to the motive force or energy (which is produced by the basic particles) required for various functional processes. Since *qi* is invisible, and what can be perceived is the result of energy, *qi* often connotes the activity itself. For example, deficiency of the *kidney qi* means deficiency of the energy required for functional processes of the *kidney*; it actually implies hypofunction of the *kidney*.

The physiological *qi* can be divided into the inborn source and the acquired source. The inborn *qi* is the innate vital essence stored in the *kidney* which was inherited from the parents; the acquired *qi* is a combination of the essence absorbed by the *spleen* from food and fresh air which is inhaled by the *lung*. These two together constitute the genuine *qi* (or vital energy), circulating in the body to each organ and tissue.

The meridians and collaterals are the passage ways along which the *qi* circulates. As they are distributed all over the body, coordination of various functional processes are realized through the *qi*. Acupuncture and moxibustion rely on this relationship between the *qi* and the meridians for successful therapy.

2. Blood

Blood is produced from the food essence absorbed by the *spleen*. The *kidney* is also closely related to the production of blood, as the *kidney* provides vital essence for bone marrow.

Blood carries nutrients through the vessels. Circulation is promoted by the *heart* with the help of the *lung*, controlled by the *spleen* which keeps the blood flowing within the vessels, and regulated by the *liver* which serves as a reservoir for blood. Deficiency of blood, a term commonly used in traditional Chinese medicine, does not necessarily mean anemia; it may also mean ischemia.

3. Vital essence

Vital essence can be divided into two categories. Congenital essence is responsible for reproduction and is called "reproductive essence." It is stored in the *kidney* and serves as the origin of life. Acquired essence is produced from nutrients in food and distributed to various organs and tissues. It serves as the material basis for life activities. Traditional Chinese medicine has it that congenital essence can be transformed into acquired essence, and acquired essence into reproductive essence after adolescence. Sexual over-indulgence is taken as an important cause of disease because it consumes the reproductive essence stored in the *kidney*, thus impairing the other organs.

4. Body fluid

Formation, distribution and excretion of body fluid (water metabolism) can be described as follows: When food and drink are digested in the stomach and intestines, the essential fluid is absorbed and transported by the *spleen* to the *heart* and *lung*. The residue, normally containing a small amount of water, is excreted in the form of feces. Essential fluid is distributed through the *heart* and *lung* to various organs and tissues all over the body. The *kidney* excretes surplus fluid as urine, and part may be excreted as sweat through the pores.

Accumulation of excessive fluid is usually due to: (1) diminished function of the *spleen* which impairs normal distribution of body fluid;

(2) diminished function of the *kidney* which causes reduced excretion of urine; and (3) impaired function of the *lung*, which usually helps with distribution of water, especially its downward flow.

Cause of Disease

The body is regarded both as a whole organism with the various parts closely related to each other and as an organic unit which adapts to the environment. Health implies harmonious coordination among the various parts of the body and adaptation to the physical environment. When normal coordination and adaptation break down, illness occurs. Thus, the fundamental mechanism of disease is the breakdown of relative equilibrium within the organism or between the organism and its environment. In traditional medical terms, this is called an imbalance of *yin* and *yang*. Medical treatment is thus aimed at restoration of normal equilibrium, bringing *yin-yang* back into balance.

Generally speaking, an imbalance of *yin-yang* is due to pathogenic factors, either originating in the external environment or evolving within the human body. With any disease, there are pathogenic factors on the one hand, and a genuine energy in the human body that resists those factors on the other. Disease is thus considered a struggle of genuine energy against pathogenic factors. Genuine energy here refers to the functioning of the organs and tissues, the adaptability of the human being to the environment, and the body's resistance to the pathogenic factors. It denotes all body functions that maintain a normal level of health.

A prominent feature of traditional Chinese medicine is the significance of genuine energy in the genesis and development of disease. As stated in *Canon of Medicine*, "When there is abundant genuine energy in the body, invasion of pathogenic factor is impossible." "A pathogenic factor such as wind, rain, cold or heat is unable to cause damage unless there is insufficient genuine energy. That is why some people with good resistance, though caught in heavy rain or strong wind, will not get ill. A pathogenic factor alone is not enough to cause disease."

Research in traditional Chinese medicine did not discover pathogens such as bacteria and viruses; pathogenic factors were rather determined by observation and analysis of clinical manifestations in the light of ancient Chinese philosophy. This made for a unique etiology, which, though not entirely logical from the modern point of view, was useful in clinical practice for its association with the therapeutic effects.

Pathogenic factors are classified into two main groups: exogenous and endogenous. Exogenous pathogenic factors encompass atmospheric changes, pestilential pathogens and trauma. The diseases caused by these factors are called exogenous diseases or external affections. Endogenous pathogenic factors are generally emotional factors (joy, anger, melancholy, anxiety, grief, fear and fright), improper diet, fatigue and over-indulgence in sex. The diseases caused by endogenous pathogenic factors are called endogenous diseases or internal injuries.

Abnormal atmospheric changes refer not only to seasonal diseases such as colds in winter and heat-stroke in summer, but also to various infectious diseases. The six kinds of atmospheric changes are: wind, cold, heat, dampness, dryness and fire (intense heat). Clinical study rather than searching for the pathogenic factors themselves determines the cause of a disease. For instance, if the diagnosis is "invasion of wind" or "wind syndrome," it does not necessarily mean that the patient was caught in a draught. The diagnosis of "wind" may encompass all those characteristics similar to an encounter with natural wind.

Wind in nature is air in motion. Rising and falling intermittently, it is usually stronger at the top of a mountain than at the base and causes the branches of a tree to sway. Diseases with the following characteristics are believed to be caused by wind and thus classified as wind syndromes.

(1) Diseases which strike suddenly and disappear in a short period of time, such as urticaria (*feng zhen*, or "wind-rash"; *feng* means wind, *zhen* means rash).

(2) Diseases with lesions constantly shifting location, such as rheumatic arthritis with migratory joint pain (*feng bi*, or "windy arthritis").

(3) General disease with symptoms centered at the top of the body, particularly the head and face, such as acute nephritis with puffy eyelids (*feng shui*, "windy edema").

(4) Aversion to wind, such as mild colds (*shang feng*, or "catching wind").

As mentioned above, the wind syndromes are classified into two categories: exogenous wind syndromes (such as colds and acute rheumatic arthritis after exposure to wind and cold) and endogenous wind syndromes (such as vertigo and stroke). It seems illogical to determine the cause of a disease based on the similarity between clinical manifestation and the natural wind. But as this kind of "etiological classification" is based on therapeutic effects, it is actually a very practical method. Colds ("catching wind"), urticaria ("wind-rash"), rheumatic arthritis with migratory pain ("windy arthritis") and acute nephritis with edema of the eyelids ("windy edema") can all be satisfactorily treated with "wind-dispelling drugs" such as Herba Schizonepetae (schizonepeta), Radix Ledebouriellae (ledebouriella root), and Herba Ephedrae (ephedra). These herbal drugs are called "wind-dispelling" for their effectiveness in treating those diseases believed to result from invasion of "exogenous wind." A single group of herbal drugs can be used to treat all those diseases with common pathogenesis.

The above analysis is applicable in the diagnosis of other atmospheric factors. Wind, cold, heat, dampness, dryness, and fire are both the categories of pathogenic factors, as well as the names of pathologic changes and their syndromes.

In endogenous diseases, determination of the pathogenic factor is necessary for the doctor to give proper advice, but diagnosis of the pathologic changes is even more important to help the patient recover from internal injuries. Pathologic changes in endogenous diseases may be similar to those of the exogenous diseases: wind, cold, heat, dampness, dryness, and fire. Stroke, for example, is usually characterized by fainting and loss of consciousness, deviation of the eyes and mouth, and hemiplegia. There is also abruptness and involuntary movement, as the distorted face or figure looks like a tree tilting in the wind. Stroke is thus called *zhong feng* (wind-stroke) in traditional Chinese medicine. There are two types of such wind syndromes, one due to exogenous wind, the other due to endogenous wind. Endogenous wind is a pathological product of dysfunctioning visceral organs caused by emotional disturbances, overfatigue or improper diet. In that it may result in a clinical syndrome, it can be taken as a pathogenic factor.

Similar conditions occur with cold, heat, dampness, dryness, and fire. These exogenous pathogenic factors originate in the external environment, but may also be created in the body, thus working as endogenous pathogenic factors. Summer heat and toxic heat are the exceptions. Always exogenous, the former refers to high external temperature, and the latter to a virulence of pathogens that cause high fever and other toxic symptoms.

Determination of the six categories of pathogenic factors can be summarized as follows:

1. Wind. Diseases caused by exogenous wind are characterized by the following: (1) sudden onset and quick subsidence; (2) lesions constantly shifting location; (3) aversion to wind. Skin diseases caused by wind are marked by itching.

Diseases caused by endogenous wind are characterized by involuntary movement such as tremor, twitching or convulsion; or the feeling of abnormal movement such as vertigo and fainting.

2. Cold. Diseases caused by exogenous cold are characterized by the following: (1) a chill or aversion to cold with cold limbs, which can hardly be alleviated by warming; (2) contraction of muscles; (3) localized pain which is aggravated by exposure to cold.

Diseases caused by endogenous cold are also marked by a chill or aversion to cold with cold limbs, but the chill can be alleviated by warming.

3. Dampness. Diseases caused by exogenous dampness display the following clinical features: (1) lingering illness; (2) heaviness in the body and limbs, or headache as if the head were tightly bound; (3) turbid discharge such as excessive leukorrhea, turbid urine, exudation from skin lesions; (4) sensation of fullness or distention due to impediment of the normal flow of *qi*; (5) loss of appetite, nausea, vomiting, and loose stools due to impairment of the digestive system.

Diseases caused by endogenous dampness are manifested by abdominal distention, loss of appetite, loose stools, white greasy tongue coating, and edema. They usually occur in those with dysfunction of the *spleen*.

4. Dryness. Diseases caused by dryness are characterized by a dry mouth, dry nose, dry throat, and dry cough.

5. Heat. Diseases caused by exogenous heat are marked by fever, thirst, scanty concentrated urine, constipation, reddened tongue with yellow coating and rapid pulse.

Diseases caused by endogenous heat are often marked by a low fever in the afternoon, a feeling of heat in the palms and soles, malar flush, night sweating, constipation, concentrated urine, reddened tongue with scanty or no coating, and thready rapid pulse.

6. Fire. Diseases caused by exogenous fire are marked by: (1) acute inflammation and localized redness, swelling, heat and pain; (2) fever, restlessness, thirst, foul breath, bitterness in the mouth, ulceration

of the tongue, and constipation; (3) bleeding such as epistaxis, hematuria, hematochezia; (4) a dark red tongue with a yellow, prickly coating, and rapid replete pulse.

Diseases caused by endogenous fire are similar to those caused by endogenous heat, but may be accompanied by irritability and insomnia.

There are, apart from the above, some other pathological products that give rise to clinical syndromes, and so are regarded as pathogenic factors, or intermediate pathogenetic factors. They are stagnated *qi* and blood, retained fluid, and accumulated phlegm. These products of dysfunctioning visceral organs, occurring in either exogenous affections or endogenous injuries, can also lead to clinical syndromes.

Stagnation of *qi* may produce a variety of syndromes marked by pain. It is generally recognized in traditional Chinese medicine that "wherever there is obstruction, there is pain." This pain is often accompanied by distention and not fixed in location. In addition, as *qi* is the energy required for the functional processes of organs, stagnation of *qi* in a certain organ may lead to a functional disturbance in that organ. Examples of this are irascibility when the *qi* is stagnated in the *liver* and constipation when *qi* is stagnated in the large intestine.

Blood stasis can also lead to further disorders as a pathogenic factor. In Western medicine, blood stasis usually refers to venous congestion, but in traditional Chinese medicine, it covers a large variety of pathological changes associated with retardation or stoppage of blood flow. The most typical case of blood stasis is extravasation, in which the blood stops flowing. Blood stasis also includes congestion, thrombosis, ischemia, and mass formation (such as enlarged liver and spleen, and tumors).

Blood stasis is usually accompanied by pain, but this pain is different from that due to stagnation of *qi*. The former is generally severe, stabbing, and fixed in location. A purplish tongue or purple spots on the tongue is often seen in patients with blood stasis.

Retention of excessive fluid is often the result of a dysfunctioning *kidney*, *spleen* or *lung*. It may produce other disorders such as vomiting (when the fluid is retained in the stomach), cough and dyspnea with thin expectoration (when it impairs the *lung*), palpitation, shortness of breath and orthopnea (when it impairs the *heart*). In all cases, the key step is to eliminate excessive fluid.

Phlegm in traditional Chinese medicine is not only the semi-fluid visible substance formed in the respiratory passages. This is called "visible phlegm" or "respiratory phlegm." In respiratory disease, although "visible phlegm" is a pathological product, it is often believed to be the cause of other symptoms such as cough and dyspnea. The key point in relieving cough and dyspnea is to dispel the phlegm.

There is also "invisible phlegm," which is supposed to cause a variety of syndromes, including some psychotic diseases (regarded as disturbance of the brain by phlegm), numbness or even hemiplegia (regarded as blocking of the meridians and collaterals by phlegm), and palpable enlarged lymph nodes (regarded as subcutaneous retention of phlegm). Though taken from the point of Western medicine, it is difficult to see why these diseases are attributed to phlegm, but in fact, all may be treated with the same phlegm dispelling therapy.

Differentiation of Syndromes

In traditional Chinese medicine, differentiation of syndromes is often more important than diagnosis of diseases. The former is based upon an overall analysis of symptoms and signs, including cause, nature and location of the illness as well as the confrontation between pathogenic factors and the body resistance. "Syndrome," in its traditional sense is not a simple summation of symptoms and signs; it rather reflects the pathogenesis and pathophysiology of a given case.

All syndromes can be classified into two or three main categories:

1. Deficiency syndromes (syndromes with a deficiency of vital capacity), in which there is insufficient body resistance, diminished functional processes, or deficiency of essential substances.

2. Excess syndromes (syndromes with an excess of pathogenic factors).

3. Syndromes with a combination of deficiency and excess, in which there is a deficiency of vital capacity and excess of pathogenic factors.

Deficiency syndromes can be divided into four groups: deficiency of *qi*, blood, *yin,* and *yang*.

Deficiency of *qi* is marked by diminished functions of various visceral organs or systems as well as lowered body resistance. The common clinical manifestations are lassitude, listlessness, feeble voice, spontaneous sweating, pallid complexion, pale tongue, and weak pulse. In addition, there is often evidence of diminished function of certain visceral organs, such as palpitation and shortness of breath aggravated by exertion (when the *heart* is chiefly involved); loss of appetite, abdominal distention and loose stools (when the *spleen* is chiefly involved).

Deficiency of blood is generally marked by pallor, pale tongue and thready pulse. There may be anemia, but if it is severe, resulting in shortness of breath, lack of strength and listlessness, it is usually diagnosed as deficiency of both *qi* and blood. Treatment in such cases should be to replenish both the *qi* and blood.

Deficiency of *yin* includes deficiency of the essence, of body fluids and of other essential substances. Deficiency of blood is a part of deficiency of *yin*, but often referred to separately to stress its significance.

General manifestations of *yin* deficiency are emaciation, dryness of the mouth and throat, scanty urine, constipation, scanty tongue coating and thready pulse. *Yin* being related to *yang*, deficiency of *yin* usually leads to a corresponding preponderance of *yang*, which may result in endogenous heat. *Yin* deficiency is often accompanied by a sensation of heat in the palms and soles, malar flush or even low fever, night sweating, reddened tongue and thready rapid pulse.

When a specific visceral organ is involved in *yin* deficiency, symptoms indicate impairment of that organ. For instance, if the *heart* is involved, insomnia and dream-disturbed sleep will result; if the *liver* is involved, there will be dizziness, tinnitus, or menstrual disorders for women; if the *lung* is involved, there will be dry cough or hoarseness; if the *kidney* is involved, lower back pain, seminal emission, sterility or infertility will result.

Deficiency of *yang* is a lack of dynamic energy needed for physiological processes, which is both a deficiency of *qi* (resulting in hypofunction of visceral organs), and deficiency of heat energy for metabolism (resulting in "cold" manifestations such as intolerance to cold). In most cases, clinical evidence of *yang* deficiency can be formulated as manifestations of *qi* deficiency plus endogenous cold, which is manifested by aversion to cold or symptoms aggravated by cold.

Excess syndromes are usually classified according to the specific pathogenic factors: wind syndromes, cold syndromes, heat syndromes, dampness syndromes, dryness syndromes, fire syndromes, phlegm syndromes, syndromes of *qi* stagnation, and syndromes of blood stasis.

The means to determine these factors was discussed in the preceding section. When a specific organ is involved other symptoms may appear. For instance, fire syndrome of the *heart* is marked by restlessness, insomnia and ulceration at the tip of the tongue; blood stasis of the *heart* is marked by angina pectoris. Fire syndrome of the *liver* is marked by headache, dizziness, irascibility, hypochondriac pain, epistaxis, or hematemesis. Wind syndrome of the *liver* is marked by tremor, twitching, spasm or even convulsion. Damp-heat of the large intestine leads to acute dysentery with discharge of mucus and blood; damp-heat of the urinary bladder leads to urinary infection with painful urination and discharge of turbid or bloody urine.

The above syndrome diagnosis is applicable for nearly all but those with acute fever. For acute febrile diseases, diagnosis will be discussed in Chapter III.

Principles of Prevention and Treatment

Disease prevention is a critical part of traditional Chinese medicine. Since disease involves two aspects, pathogenic factors and body resistance (energy that resists the pathogenic factors), both must be considered in disease prevention. Priority is usually given to building up health and strengthening body resistance. The best approach towards this end is to lead a regular life, have a proper diet, do appropriate exercise and maintain harmony in mental and emotional activities. A regular life includes adaptation to environmental changes and avoidance of overindulgence in sex and alcohol.

A secondary point is to prevent the disease from getting worse. Unaffected parts of the body should be reinforced according to the development of the disease.

Treatment is based primarily on the diagnosis of syndromes. In deficiency syndromes, the general principle of treatment is to strengthen the patient's vital capacity, which is to enhance resistance, promote the physiological processes and replenish the required substances. These approaches are called "tonification," and the drugs used, "tonics." In excess syndromes, the treatment is aimed at eliminating or dispelling the pathogenic factors. Wind-cold is thus dispelled by diaphoretics; toxic heat is reduced by heat-clearing and detoxicant drugs; dampness is removed by aromatics or diuretics; excessive fire is eliminated from the *heart* by sedatives; stagnation of *qi* is relieved by carminatives, blood stasis is eliminated by blood-activating and stasis-removing drugs.

Evaluation of a syndrome encompasses not only the cause, mechanism, location and nature of the disease, but also the struggle between the pathogenic factor and body resistance. Treatment, therefore, is not based only on the symptoms. Each patient's constitution and physical responses to the pathogenic factor are carefully considered; consequently, those with an identical disease may be treated in different ways. For example, a peptic ulcer may be diagnosed as: (1) impairment of the stomach by perverted flow of *liver qi* (in cases precipitated or aggravated by emotional upsets, manifested by epigastric pain which cannot be alleviated by food or warmth, and accompanied by belching, vomiting, acid regurgitation and the feeling of choking); (2) deficiency of the *spleen* and stomach *qi* (characterized by epigastric pain, impaired appetite and lassitude, aggravated by improper diet and alleviated by taking soft food); and (3) deficiency of the *spleen* and stomach *yang* (with the same symptoms as deficiency of the *spleen* and stomach *qi* plus aversion to cold and cold sensation in the stomach). Soothing the *liver* and harmonizing the stomach is indicated in the first case, replenishing the *spleen* and stomach *qi* in the second, and warming the *spleen* and stomach in the third.

On the other hand, different diseases may result in the same syndrome and should be treated in the same way. For example, peptic ulcer and chronic gastritis, though different pathologically, may both be diagnosed as deficiency of the *spleen* and stomach *yang*. The same warming-up therapy should therefore be applied.

In summary, it can be seen that in most cases, a doctor practicing traditional Chinese medicine treats the patient rather than the disease.

CHAPTER II
IMMUNITY IN TRADITIONAL CHINESE MEDICINE

Brief Historical Review

Immunity in the Chinese language is *mian yi*, of which *mian* means "to exempt from," and *yi* means "epidemic diseases." The term *mian yi* first appeared in Chinese medical literature in the 18th century in the book *Mian Yi Lei Fang* (*Classified Prescriptions for Exemption from Epidemic Diseases*). However, the concept can be found in *Canon of Medicine*, written 2,000 years ago. "If the human body is full of genuine energy, it will not be invaded by pathogens." "An experienced doctor would rather treat a patient with a potential disease than a patient who has already fallen ill." These statements emphasize the importance of "genuine energy" and prevention of disease. The term "genuine energy" here can be defined as the capacity to maintain normal physical functioning and resist against pathogens, including functions of immunity.

Original constitution is closely related to immunity. Traditional Chinese medicine attaches great importance to original constitution and holds that some diseases are attributed to a particular diathesis. For instance, in *Zhu Bing Yuan Hou Zong Lun* (*General Treatise on the Etiology and Symptomatology of Diseases*) paint dermatitis was regarded as a diathetic disorder.

A deficiency of genuine energy may result in a large variety of diseases. In *Yi Zong Bi Du* (*Required Readings for Medical Professionals*) compiled in 1637, the genesis of tumors was attributed to deficiency of vital energy, and therapy to reinforce this energy was recommended as treatment.

Artificial immunization was first developed by traditional Chinese medicine. Some 1,500 years ago, it was recorded in *Zhou Hou Bei Ji Fang* (*A Handbook of Prescriptions for Emergencies*) that rabies could be prevented and treated by application of dried powder from an infected dog to the bite. One of the most notable achievements in the history of traditional Chinese medicine was the invention of variolation or inoculation to prevent smallpox. Though the exact date when this method was initiated is difficult to ascertain, it was already widely used in the 16th century, hundreds of years before Jenner's cowpox inoculation of 1796. Doctors were sent from Tsarist Russia to Beijing (Peking) to learn the method in 1688. It was later introduced to Turkey and Europe.

After a long standstill, knowledge about immunity has recently leapt forward, particularly due to modern research of the traditional medical base. The following conclusions have been drawn: (1) In many patients diagnosed with deficiency syndromes, the immune function is impaired. (2) Therapies to reinforce the genuine energy can restore the normal immune function. (3) Other therapies such as heat-clearing and detoxicating, blood-activating and stasis-eliminating, and purging have an effect on immunity. (4) Some medicinal herbs are immunopotentiators, some are immunosuppressors, and some are immunomodulators.

Theoretical Aspect of Immunity in Traditional Chinese Medicine

Immunity in traditional Chinese medicine has a dual meaning: In a narrow sense, it refers to exemption from epidemic diseases, while more broadly, it means the prevention of any disease through genuine energy. Preservation and consolidation of the genuine energy thus plays an important role in preventive medicine. In clinical therapeutics, the tonification therapy (i.e., to supplement essential substances and strengthen body resistance) is widely used to treat various deficiency syndromes; and care must be taken with elimination therapies (i.e., to eliminate various pathogens) to avoid impairment of the genuine energy.

This so-called genuine energy refers to all kinds of resistance against disease, including the immunological functions. Traditional classification of genuine energy is as follows:

1. Defensive Energy or Superficial Genuine Energy

Defensive energy or superficial genuine energy serves as the first level of protection against disease. It is provided by the epithelial and epidermal barriers, among which, according to traditional Chinese medicine, the sweat pores play an important role. Adapting to changes in the external environment, they open to release sweat when the weather is hot, and close to stop it when the weather is cold. Impaired function of the pores weakens defense capability and exposes the patient to infection. This energy includes resistant mechanisms at the initial stage of an infectious disease. The confrontation of defensive energy against the invading pathogens causes a series of clinical manifestations known as "exterior syndrome" (i.e., the host response to infection at an early stage).

This is especially important in the treatment of an infectious disease with exterior syndrome. The syndrome is characterized by chills, fever, thin tongue coating and floating pulse. If there is no sweating, diaphoretics are usually indicated; if there is sweating, non-diaphoretic antipyretics are preferred. If there is sweating with the chills and fever, and the superficial defensive energy is extremely deficient, reinforcing the genuine energy is called for.

Recent studies have shown that in patients with deficient genuine energy, nonspecific immunologic functions, both cellular and humoral, are lowered. This so-called defensive energy thus encompasses immunologic functions. Pharmacological studies on medicinal herbs used for reinforcing genuine energy have also revealed that most of these herbs are immunoenhancing. This issue will be taken up later in the chapter.

2. Genuine Energy of the Visceral Organs

The genuine energy of the visceral organs is that portion of energy required to maintain normal functioning of these organs. Each visceral organ has its own genuine energy. As described in Chapter I, visceral organs are the core structures and systems responsible for vital functions of the body. The collective genuine energy of these organs is responsible for all human vital activities. The *spleen* and *kidney* are the two most closely associated with the production of genuine energy, which is formed by a combination of inborn (inherited) and acquired vital energy. "The *kidney* is the foundation of the inborn constitution"; inborn vital energy originates therein. "The *spleen* determines the acquired constitution, providing the material basis for acquired vital energy." Diminished function of either the *kidney* or the *spleen* will lead to deficiency of the genuine energy.

In recent years, immunological changes in patients with hypofunction of the *spleen* or *kidney* have been studied extensively. Results from different studies are consistent: In patients with hypofunction of the *spleen,* both cellular and humoral immunity are decreased (as shown by decreased peripheral blood lymphocyte count, weakened response to phyto-hemagglutinin, lowered T lymphocyte ratio, reduced lymphocyte transformation rate, depressed E rosette forming rate, and lowered serum immunoglobulin A and G levels). Herbal treatment to reinforce the *spleen* tends to return the above indices to normal.

In patients with hypofunction of the *kidney*, immunologic functions are usually more markedly impaired than in those with hypofunction of the *spleen*, especially when these two conditions are compared in patients suffering from the same disease (e.g., chronic bronchitis). Improvement of immunologic functions has also been observed after *kidney*-tonifying treatment.

On the other hand, although the immune function is one of the mechanisms of tissue defense, immune reactions which trigger inflammation can be amplified to a level recognizable as an immunologically mediated disease. For example, bronchial asthma may be IgE-mediated. In a report by Shanghai Medical University, increased serum immunoglobulin E (IgE) and decreased suppressor T cells (Ts) were found in chronic asthmatics with *kidney* hypofunction. Treatment with *kidney*-tonifying therapy suppressed serum IgE and increased T cells.

3. Genuine Energy of the Meridians

The meridians and collaterals form a system to connect parts of the body into an organic whole and keep them in a physiologic state of coordination. Genuine energy of the meridians is important for homeostasis and regulation of various processes. This is the basis of acupuncture, which aims to regulate body functions through stimulation of genuine energy of the meridians. Further discussion on this point will be made in Chapter VII.

Stimulation of genuine energy of the meridians to regulate functional processes also regulates immune functions. Acupuncture has a marked effect on peripheral white blood cells, phagocytosis of macrophages, serum complement and immunoglobulin levels. The therapeutic effect of acupuncture in the treatment of infectious diseases, such as epidemic encephalitis B and acute bacillary dysentery, is attributed to the action on the patient's immune system. The serum level of lysozyme (an enzyme that destroys bacteria by attacking their cell walls), for example, increases markedly during acupuncture therapy.

Medicinal Herbs and Immunity

1. Herbal Immunopotentiators

A number of medicinal herbs used in traditional Chinese medicine enhance the immune response. This may be an increase in the rate at which the immune response develops, an increase in the intensity or level of the response, or a prolongation of the response. These herbs may act on cellular (cell-mediated) immunity, on humoral immunity, or on both.

(1) Cellular-immunity herbs

Cellular immunity is one of the chief protective functions of the human body. T cells are the primary effectors of cellular immunity; subsets of T cells maturing into cytotoxic cells can cause lysis of virus-infected or foreign cells. Other non-specific immune cells such as neutrophils and reticulo-endothelial cells are also involved in cellular immunity. The following work to enhance cellular immunity: *qi*-tonics such as Radix Ginseng (ginseng), Radix Astragali (astragalus root), Radix Codonopsis Pilosulae (pilose asiabell root) and Rhizoma Atractylodis Macrocephalae (white atractylodes rhizome); *yin*-tonics such as Fructus Corni (dogwood fruit), Fructus Ligustri Lucidi (lucid ligustrum fruit), Plastrum Testudinis (tortoise plastron) and Carapax Trionycis (turtle shell); heat-clearing and detoxifying herbs such as Rhizoma Coptidis (coptis root), Radix Scutellariae (scutellaria root), Herba Oldenlandiae (oldenlandia) and Flos Lonicerae (honeysuckle flower) and blood-activating herbs such as Radix Salviae Miltiorrhizae (red sage root), Rhizoma Ligustici Chuanxiong (chuanxiong rhizome), Rhizoma Sparganii (burreed tuber) and Rhizoma Zedoariae (zedoary).

Different herbs enhance cellular immunity through different routes. For example, Radix Codonopsis Pilosulae (pilose asiabell root) and Rhizoma Atractylodis Macrocephalae (white atractylodes rhizome) increase the T cell ratio; Radix Ginseng (ginseng), Rhizoma Atractylodis Macrocephalae (white atractylodes rhizome), radix Salviae Miltiorrhizae (red sage root), Rhizoma Ligustici Chuanxiong (chuanxiong rhizome) and many heat-clearing and detoxifying herbs promote lymphocyte transformation; Radix Ginseng (ginseng), Radix Astragali (astragalus root) and Fructus Ligustri Lucidi (lucid ligustrum fruit) increase blood polymorphonuclear cells (also called microphages for their phagocytic action); Radix Ginseng (ginseng), Radix Astragali (astragalus root) and Radix Codonopsis Pilosulae (pilose asiabell root) promote the phagocytic action of mononuclear macrophages. All the herbs listed above, particularly those for heat-clearing and detoxifying, promote the phagocytic action of reticulo-endothelial cells.

(2) Humoral-immunity herbs

Humoral immunity refers primarily to antibodies. Antibodies are a kind of immunoglobulin synthesized and secreted by plasma cells maturing from B lymphocyte precursors present in all lymphoid tissue except the thymus. Herbs activating humoral immunity are mostly tonics such as Radix Astragali (astragalus root), Radix Ginseng (ginseng), Radix Codonopsis Pilosulae (pilose asiabell root), Semen Cuscutae (dodder seed), Ganoderma Lucidum (lucid ganoderma) and Radix Rehmanniae (rehmannia root). Many non-specific immune factors such as complements, lysozyme, properdin and interferon are also involved in humoral immunity. Radix Astragali (astragalus root) promotes induction of interferon during viral infection. *Xianggu* mushroom is an activator of complement 3. Radix Ginseng (ginseng) and Radix Astragali (astragalus root) augment the production of antibodies. Radix Rehmanniae (rehmannia root), Radix Astragali (astragalus root) and *Xianggu* mushroom increase the serum IgG level, and Radix Astragali (astragalus root) and Ganoderma Lucidum (lucid ganoderma) increase the IgA and IgM levels.

From the above, it can be seen that of the many herbs used to enhance the immune response, Radix Astragali (astragalus root) stands out.

The function of Radix Astragali has been studied extensively with the following results: It promotes lymphocyte transformation in humans and proliferation of rosette-forming cells in immunized mice. It acts to increase the phagocytosis of reticulo-endothelial cells comparable to that of BCG. The Institute of Epidemic Diseases in the Chinese Academy of Medical Sciences also found that administration of this herbal medicine enhanced leukocyte induction of interferon and increased immunoglobulin A and G in the nasal secretion of subjects vulnerable to influenza. This drug has also been used to prevent influenza, especially with those who have suffered from repeated attacks.

That Radix Astragali promotes interferon induction is a recent discovery, but use of the root to protect against influenza can be dated to ancient times. *Shen Nong's Herbal* lists Radix Astragali as a superior tonic (a tonic that can be used for a long time without adverse effects). In the 14th century a well-known formula called *Yu Ping Feng San* (Jade-Screen Powder) composed principally of Radix Astragali, in combination with Rhizoma Atractylodis Macrocephalae and Radix Ledebouriellae, was initiated to reinforce the genuine energy so as to strengthen superficial physical resistance and arrest excessive spontaneous sweating. This formula was particularly effective against repeated colds or influenza for patients with insufficient genuine energy. A cold, in the Chinese language, is expressed as "attack by draughts." This *Yu Ping Feng San* (Jade-Screen Powder) was like a screen used to shield off draughts. The formula is still used widely, with particular success in preventing colds or influenza in patients with chronic nephritis.

Radix Ginseng (ginseng) is another herb which is probably even more popular than Radix Astragali (astragalus root). Recorded in *Shen Nong's Herbal* as a superior tonic, it has been widely used for reinforcing genuine energy, even in cases of prostration. It should be noted that different species of Radix Ginseng (ginseng) have different pharmacological actions. In *Shen Nong's Herbal*, Radix Ginseng (ginseng) refers to the dried root of Panax ginseng C. A. May, which grows primarily in the northeast of China and is taken as a *qi*-tonic to reinforce genuine energy. American ginseng refers to the dried root of Panax quinquefolium L, which grows in the United States, Canada, and France and is taken as a *yin*-tonic to promote fluid secretion.

Radix Ginseng (ginseng) has been studied extensively in China and other countries. The immunopharmacological actions can be summarized as follows: It enhances immune surveillance in cancer patients, increases peripheral white blood cells and prevents leukopenia during chemotherapy. It promotes lymphocyte transformation in healthy bodies, and helps prevent influenza and other upper respiratory infections.

It has also been shown in animal experiments that intravenous or oral administration of ginsenoside, a saponin derived from Radix Ginseng (ginseng), increases phagocytosis of the reticulo endothelial system and counteracts inhibition of macrophages induced by cortisone or endotoxins. Oral administration of the polysaccharide derived from Radix Ginseng (ginseng) also remarkably increases phagocytosis of the reticulo-endothelial system. Furthermore, both the saponin and polysaccharide of Radix Ginseng (ginseng) elevate the serum complement level and promote production of antibodies and hemolysin.

Radix Codonopsis Pilosulae (pilose asiabell root), of a lesser potency, can be used in place of Radix Ginseng (ginseng). Like Radix Ginseng (ginseng), it increases phagocytosis of the reticulo-endothelial system and counteracts inhibition of macrophages induced by cortisone and endotoxins.

2. Herbal Immunosuppressors

Under normal circumstances, a well-controlled immune response protects the host from invading antigens. However, a regulatory defect in the host defense system may damage tissue and result in disease. Immune-mediated damage can be divided into the following types: type I— allergic reactions (IgE-mediated); type II— cytotoxic reactions of antibodies (IgM- or IgG-mediated); type III— immune complex formation (IgG-, IgM-, IgA-mediated); type IV— delayed hypersensitivity; and autoimmune diseases. In all the above, suppression of the immune response is indicated.

(1) Allergic reaction (type I)

In this reaction, a mediator release is triggered by antigen interaction with IgE. Mediators such as histamine, SRS-A (slow reacting substance of anaphylaxis) and bradykinin released from mast cells and basophils are responsible for allergic reactions. These reactions are: an increase in vascular permeability, contraction of the smooth muscles of the skin and respiratory tracts, local hyperemia, edema and increased glandular secretion (as in urticaria, bronchial asthma, allergic rhinitis, and other allergic diseases). Herbal treatment works with all of the above.

According to traditional medical theory, some allergies are classified as "wind syndromes" because of their sudden onset and abrupt subsidence, as discussed in Chapter I. Herbs effective for these diseases are called "wind-dispelling" drugs. Wind-dispelling herbs commonly used for allergic diseases are Herba Ephedrae (ephedra), Ramulus Cinnamomi (cinnamon twigs), Radix Ledebouriellae (ledebouriella root), Flos Magnoliae (magnolia), Fructus Xanthii (cocklebur fruit), and Radix Bupleuri (bupleurum root).

According to modern research, herbs in this category often inhibit the release of mediators to act against allergic reactions. But this is not their only anti-allergic action. Fructus Xanthii (xanthium fruit), Herba Ephedrae (ephedra) and Cortex Cinnamomi (cinnamon bark) also elevate serum IgG level to neutralize allergen and increase the T cell ratio to inhibit the production of IgE. Besides the "wind-dispelling" drugs, many other herbs may be used to counteract allergic reactions. Ganoderma Lucidum (lucid ganoderma), Herba Epimedii (epimedium) and Fructus Psoraleae (psoralea fruit) relieve bronchial spasm caused by histamine. That is why these tonics can be used to treat chronic bronchitis and bronchial asthma. Radix Scutellariae (scutellaria root) inhibits the release of histamine and SRS-A. Radix Sophorae Flavescentis (flavescent sophora root) is an effective drug for treating allergic dermatitis and eczema. Laboratory studies have revealed that it increases intracellular content of cAMP by inhibiting phosphodiesterase and thus prevents the mast cells from releasing the biologically active substances as mediators.

(2) Cytotoxic reactions of antibodies (type II)

In this kind of reaction, antibodies against normal cells or tissues bind complements and initiate a sequence of events resulting in cell lysis of tissue injury. Examples of type II antibody-mediated cytotoxic reactions include red cell lysis in transfusion reactions, autoimmune hemolytic anemia, drug-induced hemolytic anemia, idiopathic thrombocytopenic purpura, and some cases of granulocytopenia. Some of the blood-activating herbs such as Radix Angelicae Sinensis (Chinese angelica root), Radix Salviae Miltiorrhizae (red sage root) and Herba Leonuri (motherwort), that inhibit complete and incomplete antibodies of IgM and IgG, work against this reaction. Besides these drugs, Fructus Amomi (amomum fruit) has also been found to have inhibitory action on immunological hemolytic reaction.

(3) Immune complex formation (type III)

Clearance of antigens by immune complex formation is a highly effective mechanism of host defense. After antigen exposure, certain soluble antigen-antibody complexes circulate, and if not cleared by the reticuloendothelial system, can be deposited in blood vessel walls, renal glomeruli, and other tissues. Immune-complex diseases include glomurulonephritis, rheumatoid arthritis, systemic lupus erythematosis, and scleroderma.

Heat-clearing and detoxifying herbs such as Herba Oldenlandiae (oldenlandia), Flos Lonicerae (honeysuckle flower) and Fructus Forsythiae (forsythia fruit) and wind-dispelling herbs such as Herba Ephedrae (ephedra), Folium Perillae (perilla leaf) work to reduce the antigen-antibody complex reaction by eliminating antigens. Astragalus root has some inhibitory effect on the antigen-antibody complex reaction. A large dose of Radix Astragali (astragalus root) may have some effect in treating nephritis, as nephritic rats treated with the root were found to have milder albuminuria and less kidney pathology than those untreated.

(4) Delayed hypersensitivity reactions (type IV)

Inflammatory reactions initiated by mononuclear leukocytes and not by antibodies alone are called delayed hypersensitivity reactions. A "delayed" reaction is that in which a secondary cellular response occurs 24 to 48 hours or more after antigen exposure; an "immediate" hypersensitivity reaction generally occurs within 12 hours of the antigen challenge and is initiated by basophils mediator release or a preformed antibody. Delayed hypersensitivity may occur in contact dermatitis, chronic hepatitis B, and a homograft reaction. Since tissue damage in delayed hypersensitivity is brought about by impaired cell-mediated immunity, herbs potentiating cellular immunity are apparently important. Radix Scutellariae (scutellaria root) and Rhizoma Coptidis (coptis root) inhibit delayed hypersensitivity by enhancing the phagocytic action of white blood cells to absorb antigens. Some tonics such as Radix Astragali (astragalus root) and Fructus Lycii (wolfberry fruit) elevate the T cell ratio and strengthen the cellular immune function. They thus relieve delayed hypersensitivity reactions, particularly in the treatment of chronic hepatitis. Radix Angelicae Sinensis (Chinese angelica root) and Bombyx Batryticatus (batryticated silkworm) act against rejection of homograft.

3. Immunological Features of Herbal Therapy

Although there are exceptions, many herbs that act on the immune system can be taken as nonspecific immunomodulators. Immunopotentiators usually exert maximum effects on a suppressed immune system, and immunosuppressors suppress the immune function only when there is immune-mediated damage. Some even have bidirectional regulatory effects that enhance the immune function when it is insufficient and inhibit it when it is abnormally active. Those with bidirectional effects are sometimes called "adaptogen-like" substances. This may explain why both immunopotentiators and immunosuppressing seldom bring about adverse reactions.

The pharmacological actions of herbal immunomodulators can be classified as follows:

(1) Regulatory actions on the adrenocortex

Herbs that stimulate the pituitary-adrenocortical functions include Radix Ginseng (ginseng), Radix Codonopsis Pilosulae (pilose asiabell root), Fructus Schisandrae (schisandra fruit) and Ganoderma Lucidum (lucid ganoderma). Some herbs such as Radix Aconiti Praeparata (prepared aconite root), Radix Polygoni Multiflori (fleeceflower root) and Radix Astragali (astragalus root) have some actions similar to the adrenocortical hormone, and thus regulate the immune functions through neuro-humoral mechanisms. Rhizoma Polygonati (Siberian solomonseal rhizome), Radix Rehmanniae (rehmannia root) and Radix Glycyrrhizae (liquorice) antagonize the feedback inhibition of the adrenocortical hormone. All regulate immunity through the hypothalamo-adenopituitary-adrenocortical system.

It should be noted that Radix Ginseng (ginseng) works widely to regulate the physiological processes that normalize disordered functions. Although it has no adrenocortical hormone-like action, it simulates the adrenocortical function by increasing ACTH secretion of the hypophysis.

Radix Acanthopanacis Senticosi (acanthopanax root) can also be taken as modulator, as it both stimulates and augments the inhibition of the central nervous system. In stress reaction, it not only prevents atrophy of the thymus, but also checks shrinkage of the adrenal glands.

(2) Regulatory actions on cyclic nucleosides

Cyclic nucleosides play an important role in immunological reactions. Cyclic 3', 5'-adenosine monophosphate (cAMP) serves as a "second messenger" in the regulation of intracellular metabolism. There is a balance between cAMP and cGMP for maintaining homeostatic controls of cell activation. The antigen-induced release of histamine from basophils is repealed by agents known to raise intracellular levels of cAMP. It has also been shown that immunologic reactions, such as lymphocyte-mediated cytotoxicity and inhibition of macrophage migration, are repealed by agents which rise with cAMP levels. Radix Ginseng (ginseng) raises cAMP levels in the adrenal glands and regulates cAMP and cGMP in some organs. The effect of Radix Astragali (astragalus root) on immunity is related to its action on intracellular cAMP metabolism. Fructus Ziziphi Jujubae (Chinese date) is rich of cAMP-like substances and augments the antiasthmatic effect of ephedra and related drugs when used in combination.

(3) Regulatory actions on nucleic acids

Some herbs, particularly the tonics, promote synthesis of DNA and RNA, thus improving nucleic acid metabolism to produce more bioactive enzymes and hormones. Modulation of immune disorders by these herbs is processed through slow regulation. In experiments with animals, *yang*-tonics such as Radix Aconiti Praeparata (prepared aconite root), Cortex Cinnamomi (cinnamon bark), Semen Cuscutae (dodder seed), and Herba Epimedii (epimedium) have been shown, with the aid of isotope labeling, to raise the DNA synthetic ratio when it is low, while *yin*-tonics such as Radix Rehmanniae (rehmannia root), Radix Ophiopogonis (ophiopogon root) and Plastrum Testudinis (tortoise plastron) lower the DNA synthetic ratio when it is abnormally high.

The antibacterial action of certain herbs is due to their inhibition of nucleic acid synthesis of bacteria. Radix Coptidis (coptis root) acts to inhibit RNA synthesis of bacteria; Cortex Phellodendri (phellodendron bark) inhibits RNA synthesis; and Radix et Rhizoma Rhei (rhubarb) acts strongly to inhibit lactic dehydrogenase.

(4) Regulatory actions on T cells

T cells are thymus-derived cells that participate in a variety of cell-mediated immune reactions and in the modulation of antibody secretion of B cells. There are subsets of T cells: helper T cells and suppressor T cells. The former cooperate with B cells in antibody formation, while the latter suppress secretion of auto-antibodies. As mentioned above, many tonics improve both the quantity and the quality of T cells, so that they can modulate immune reactions.

(5) Bi-directional regulation

Some herbs exhibit a bi-directional regulatory action when the body is suffering from different disorders. For example, the above mentioned *Yu Ping Feng San* (Jade-Screen Powder) has been shown in animal experiments to increase the formation of antibodies if the immune reaction in the animal is low and decrease the formation if the immune reaction is abnormally high. Radix Coptidis (coptis root) and Herba Oldenlandiae (oldenlandia) inhibit the formation of antibodies, while at the same time promoting lymphocyte transformation, particularly in the case of weakened cellular immunity and hyperactive humoral immunity. Another common formula, *Sheng Mai San* (Pulse-Activating Powder), composed of Radix Ginseng (ginseng), Radix Ophiopogonis (ophiopogon root) and Fructus Schisandrae (schisandra fruit), has also been shown to have dual actions on immunity: it inhibits delayed hypersensitive reaction and counteracts immunosuppression caused by chemotherapy.

Herbs with such bi-directional actions of "adaptogen-like" substances, which show no action if the organism is not under stress, can restore normal processes if there are disorders due to stress or damage. These substances not only act on the immune functions, but on many others as well. Radix Ginseng (ginseng) protects the adrenocortex from hypertrophy caused by ACTH and from atrophy due to prolonged use of adrenocorticosteroids. Radix Astragali (astragalus root) raises blood pressure in hypotensive cases, and lowers it in renal hypertension.

Examples of Herbal Treatment in Diseases Related to Immune Disorders

Allergic Rhinitis (Hay Fever)

Allergic rhinitis is an example of type I allergic reaction. Characterized by sneezing, runny nose, obstruction of the nasal passages, and pharyngeal and conjunctival itching, it may be seasonal or nonseasonal. In Western countries, though seasonal allergic rhinitis is called "hay fever," the symptom complex is neither produced by hay nor associated with fever. In traditional Chinese medicine, allergic rhinitis is attributed to the attack of wind. From the modern medical perspective, it has been shown that some weeds which depend upon the wind for cross-pollination, as well as certain grasses and trees, produce enough pollen distributed by air currents to elicit seasonal allergic rhinitis. Nonseasonal or perennial allergic rhinitis may occur in response to allergens that are present in animal dander, industrial chemicals, or the dust accumulating at work or home. Apart from avoiding the offending allergen, Western treatment generally relies on immunotherapy and use of antihistamines. Though effective in some cases, immunotherapy may cause a severe adverse local or systemic reaction, antihistamines may result in drowsiness and gastro-intestinal distress.

Tianjin Institute of Integrated Traditional Chinese and Western Medicines has successfully treated 373 cases of allergic rhinitis with the following formula: Radix Astragali (astragalus root), Radix Ledebouriellae (ledebouriella root), Rhizoma Atractylodis Macrocephalae (white atractylodes rhizome), Radix Codonopsis Pilosulae (pilose asiabell root), Fructus Schisandrae (schisandra fruit), Fructus Mume (black plum), Rhizoma Acori Graminei (grass-leaved sweetflag rhizome) and Radix Curcumae (curcuma root). For seasonal allergic rhinitis or an acute attack of nonseasonal rhinitis, Flos Magnoliae (magnolia flower), Fructus Xanthii (cocklebur fruit), Herba Ephedrae (ephedra), and Herba Asari (asarum herb) were added to expel the "wind-evil" and relieve nasal obstruction. All of the 373 cases were treated with a Western antihistamine (chlorpheniramine maleate, 4 mg three times a day taken orally for two to four weeks) before the herbal treatment to be used as comparison. During the treatment with chlorpheniramine maleate, the symptoms were controlled or alleviated in 216 of the cases (57.6%), but all of them suffered a relapse two weeks after withdrawal of the drug. In addition, side effects such as drowsiness, dizziness and dryness of the mouth were experienced by 293 (78.6%) of the patients. After a one-month course of the herbal treatment, there was a marked improvement in 232 cases (62.2%): nasal itching, sneezing, nasal discharge and obstruction were eliminated, and nasal mucosa was normalized; and there was no recurrence in three months. In 78 other cases (20.9%), symptoms were alleviated, attacks reduced and the edema of nasal mucosa markedly mitigated. In only 63 cases (16.9%) did the treatment prove ineffective. Among the original 287 patients, 249 remained cured two years after the herbal treatment and 38 suffered relapses, the recurrence rate being only 13.2%.

Laboratory findings showed plasma cyclic nucleotide changes in the patients: lowered cAMP levels and cAMP/cGMP ratio and elevated cGMP level in comparison with the normal values. After herbal treatment, plasma cAMP was increased, and cGMP decreased; the cAMP/cGMP ratio thus returned to normal. It is interesting to note that in the cases treated effectively by the herbs, there were marked changes in plasma cyclic nucleotides before treatment, while in those where herbal treatment proved ineffective, the nucleotides were approximately normal beforehand. Therefore, decreased plasma cAMP, increased plasma cGMP and greatly lowered cAMP/cGMP ratio may be taken as an index for selection of cases appropriate for treatment with the above herbal formula.

ABO Hemolysis

Herbal prevention of ABO hemolytic disease in newborns can be taken as an example of traditional Chinese medical treatment of autoimmune hemolytic diseases.

During pregnancy, small amounts of fetal blood are leaked into the mother's circulatory system, this may trigger antibody formation in the mother. Particularly during delivery, when the placenta is detached, bleeding from the cord into the mother's circulation can elicit an immune response. Hemolytic disease in the newborn due to ABO incompatibility (in most cases when a Group O mother has either a Group A or B infant) occurs when the mother's antibodies against the child's blood group cross the placenta in high concentration. The most frequent signs in the newborn are anemia and rapidly developing jaundice, since the baby's hematopoieitc tissue may not be able to compensate for the increased red cell destruction and the immature liver can not conjugate enough bilirubin to be excreted with bile. As bilirubin accumulates in the plasma, it may cross the blood-brain barrier and cause damage in the form of kernicterus to the nervous system. Severe immunization causes fetal hydrops, and the fetus may die in the uterus. In these cases, if the father is homozygous for the relevant blood group, prognosis is poor for future babies. Modern treatment includes intrauterine transfusion of compatible blood during the last trimester of pregnancy if the results of amniocentesis and antibody tests indicate a serious case, exchange transfusion immediately after delivery, and phototherapy with ultraviolet light (which is only effective for mild cases).

Herbal medicine has repeatedly been proven effective for prevention and treatment of ABO hemolytic disease in the newborn. Peking Union Medical College undertook a controlled study of 24 pregnant women with a history of ABO hemolytic disease of the newborn, in which 11 were treated with preventative herbal medicine and 13 with no herbs at all. In the herbal prevention group, only mild jaundice was encountered which was cured without any other treatment. In the control group, 12 children died; the one survival case suffered from kernicterus. In a latter study, 35 pregnant women, who had delivered babies with severe jaundice and hydrops or had repeated miscarriages, were treated with herbal medicine. All were of incompatible blood groups with their husbands: 34 were Group O, and one Group A, while the husbands were Group A, B or AB. The titer of serum IgG against A or B during pregnancy was > 1:64 in all cases.

After treatment, 28 babies had no hemolytic disease and 10 had mild hemolysis. The mortality rate was 0%, though it had been 56.8% during previous pregnancies and delivery. Three to thirteen years later, all the children were developing normally. When the mothers' serum IgG was rechecked after herbal treatment, it showed marked reduction in most cases, especially in those who had non-hemolytic infants.

The herbal formula used for prevention and treatment of ABO hemolytic disease of the newborn is as follows: Herba Leonuri (motherwort) 500g, Radix Paeoniae Alba (white peony root) 180g, Radix Aucklandiae (aucklandia root) 12g, Radix Angelicae Sinensis (Chinese angelica root) 150g, and Rhizoma Ligustici Chuanxiong (chuanxiong rhizome) 500g. The above is mixed, pulverized and made into honey pills (each pill 9g). One pill is taken twice a day from the 17th week of pregnancy (or after diagnosis) until delivery.

Systemic Sclerosis

Systemic sclerosis, also called scleroderma, is a multi-system disorder of unknown etiology characterized by fibrosis of the skin, blood vessels and various visceral organs. The disease usually begins insidiously, the first symptom often being Raynaud's phenomenon. Ninety-five percent of the cases experience this phenomenon, which is episodic vasoconstriction of small arteries and arterioles of fingers, toes, and semidome at the tip of the nose and the earlobes precipitated by exposure to cold or emotional stress. Most prominent is the overproduction of collagen, which is thought to be due to aberrant regulation of fibroblast growth and increased biosythesis of connective tissue. Two subsets with some overlap can be identified. The first, referred to as progressive systemic sclerosis, is characterized by rapid symmetric skin thickening of proximal and distal extremities, the face, and trunk as well as involvement of internal organs. The second is limited to cutaneous scleroderma, which is defined by symmetric skin thickening in the fingers, distal extremities or the face.

In the development of fibrosis, immunologic mechanisms play an important role. Numerous immunologic abnormalities have been noted in patients with systemic sclerosis. Antinuclear antibodies are found in most patients and hypergammaglobulinemia in at least one-third. Systemic sclerosis is also found in association with other connective tissue diseases suspected to be of autoimmune origin.

In Western medicine, no drug therapy can cure this disease. In uncontrolled studies D-penicillamine has been reported to reduce skin thickening and prevent development of significant organ involvement. However, this drug is quite toxic; its complications include glomerulonephritis with nephrotic syndrome, aplastic anemia, leukopenia and thrombocytopenia. Other side effects are fever, rash, anorexia and nausea. Glucocorticoids may also be indicated, but again, there is a risk with long-term use.

The skin lesion of systemic sclerosis was well described in ancient Chinese literature as one of the typical manifestations of "blood stasis." In recent years this disease has been treated successfully with "stasis-eliminating" therapy. The Chinese Academy of Medical Sciences treated a group of 311 cases of systemic sclerosis with "stasis-eliminating" herbs. Disappearance or alleviation of Raynaud's phenomenon occurred in 95% of the cases along with pathological improvement. The First Medical College of Shanghai also treated 335 cases of systemic sclerosis, of which 248 were systemic and 87 limited. After one to four months, a marked effect was observed in 35.5% of the cases, as manifested by improvement of skin lesions, normalization or marked improvement of joint movement, disappearance or remarkable alleviation of Raynaud's phenomenon, as well as an obvious improvement in the general condition. The total rate of effectiveness was 92.8%. Angiographic and plethysmographic studies also showed amelioration of peripheral vascular changes.

The herbs used in the treatment were both compound prescriptions composed chiefly of Radix Salviae Miltiorrhizae (red sage root), Radix Angelicae Sinensis (Chinese angelica root), Radix Paeoniae Rubra (red peony root), Flos Carthami (safflower) and Herba Leonuri (motherwort); and single ingredients, such as an intravenous drip of extract of Radix Salviae Miltiorrhizae (red sage root) or intramuscular injection of extract of Radix Angelicae Sinensis (Chinese angelica root).

CHAPTER III
HERBS VS. INFECTIONS

Antimicrobial drugs represent one of the most important advances in modern drug therapy. The discovery of penicillin in particular has altered the outcome of infections; there are now dozens of antimicrobial agents available. Many problems, however, remain: lack of effective microbial agents for treatment of viral infections, development of antibiotic resistance in microbes, toxicity of microbial agents and allergic reaction to these agents. The most important point in this respect is that antimicrobial agents alone do not constitute full treatment for infections. To clarify this, we must first see how microbes interact with their human hosts.

There are many different microorganisms that infect the human body. The ability of a specific pathogen to cause disease depends on the interaction between its intrinsic pathogenic potential, or virulence, and the defensive capacity of the host to contain and neutralize the infectious threat. Therefore, as always in traditional Chinese medicine, both the pathogenic (microbial) factors and the condition of the host factors should be taken into account.

The virulence of a pathogen is relative; microorganisms with normally low virulence or those which normally rest latent in the host can cause severe disease when the host's defense capacity is weakened. This pathogenic potential allows the pathogen to reside, multiply, invade and destroy host tissue. The host simultaneously recruits defensive measures, particularly the immune mechanisms to contain infection. Each step in this pathogenesis is a complex interplay of microbial action and host reaction. The difference in strength between microbial virulence and host immunity determines the outcome of disease: when host defensive capacity eradicates the offending agent, resolution occurs; when host factors are evenly balanced against microbial factors, chronic infection may result; and when host responses fail to protect against microbial factors, there is dissemination of infection.

One of the characteristics of traditional herbal treatment of infections is the judgment of the balance between host and microbial factors. The prescription is usually a composite, including ingredients which act directly against the pathogen, strengthen the patient's defensive capacity, and help the patient recover from injury caused by the pathogen. In other words, these herbal medicines are prescribed to treat both the disease and the syndrome in the traditional sense.

Differentiation of Syndromes in Acute Infections

A syndrome in traditional Chinese medicine is not simply a group of symptoms. Traditional syndrome diagnosis includes determination of the cause, nature and location of the ailment as well as the condition of confrontation between the pathogenic factors and body resistance. Since acute infections are generally caused by heat pathogens (such as wind-heat, toxic heat and damp-heat) which give rise to "hot" ailments, and body resistance has not yet been badly damaged, treatment is generally localized. This may be the site where the pathological change takes place (e.g., acute dysentery is often diagnosed as damp-heat in the large intestine, and pneumonia as heat in the lung), but in most cases, location refers to the stage in the natural course of an infectious disease. It is believed in traditional Chinese medicine that acute infections are due to the invasion of external pathogens, and the outside of the body is usually attacked first. At the first stage, therefore, the infection is frequently manifested as an "exterior syndrome." The pathogens then drive into the interior of the body, causing various syndromes related to each stratum of the body which the pathological changes have involved. Generally speaking, the syndromes of acute infectious diseases fall into one of the following patterns.

1. Exterior Syndrome
This syndrome is usually encountered in the initial stage of an infectious disease when the pathogen exists in the exterior part of the body. It is characterized by fever, chills or aversion to cold, headache, a thin coating on the tongue and floating pulse. The general rule for treating this syndrome is to use diaphoretics to expel heat from the exterior portion of the body, such as Herba Schizonepetae (schizonepeta), Radix Ledebouriellae (ledebouriella root), Folium Mori (mulberry

leaf), or Flos Chrysanthemi (chrysanthemum flower).

2. Half-exterior Half-interior Syndrome

This syndrome is characterized by alternate fever and chills, fullness and a choking feeling in the chest and costal regions, bitter taste in the mouth, dry throat, nausea and loss of appetite, and taut pulse. It is so called because it is believed that the affection is located between the exterior and interior portions of the body. "Mediation" therapy is indicated, in which herbal drugs such as Radix Bupleuri (bupleurum root) and Radix Scutellariae (scutellaria root) are used.

3. Interior Syndromes

There are a number of interior syndromes which can be classified into the following patterns according to the portion or stratum of the body affected.

(1) Pattern I (involvement of the *qi* system). The *qi* system chiefly refers to the lung, stomach, intestines and gallbladder. It can be further divided into sub-patterns:

Pattern I-a: Involvement of the lung is usually manifested by high fever without chills, sweating, dire thirst, reddened tongue with yellow coating, and full and rapid pulse. Treatment should be aimed at clearing heat from the lung, the chief ingredients in the prescription being Gypsum Fibrosum (gypsum), Rhizoma Anemarrhenae (anemarrhena rhizome), and other heat-clearing and detoxifying herbs.

Pattern I-b: Involvement of the stomach and intestines is characterized by high fever (or tidal fever in the afternoon), constipation, fullness and distention of the abdomen, restlessness, yellow and dry tongue coating or prickly tongue with gray coating, and forceful pulse. Treatment should be aimed at purging the gastro-intestinal tract of accumulated heat. The principal drug for this purpose is Radix et Rhizoma Rhei (rhubarb).

(2) Pattern II (involvement of the *ying* system). The *ying* system refers to the "heart" or the central nervous system. When it is affected, there is usually high fever, restlessness, delirium, and dry crimson tongue. Treatment seeks to remove heat to cause resuscitation, Calculus Bovis (ox gallstone) is most commonly used to this end.

(3) Pattern III (involvement of the blood system). This pattern is marked by high fever, skin eruptions or bleeding (such as epistaxis or

bloody stools), deep red or purple tongue, and weak and rapid pulse. Treatment, which aims to eliminate heat from blood, relies primarily on Cornu Rhinoceri* (rhinoceros horn) and Radix Rehmanniae (rehmannia root).

The above scheme of syndrome differentiation and treatment is often used for acute infections caused by heat or, in severe cases, by toxic heat. If the infection is caused by other groups of pathogens such as damp pathogens (usually combined with heat and called damp-heat), the clinical manifestations are modified, and treatment should be altered.

Generally speaking, infections caused by damp-heat are characterized by the following additional manifestations.

Exterior syndromes: headaches as if the head were tightly bound, lassitude, white greasy coating of the tongue and soft, slippery pulse associated with chilliness and fever. Interior syndromes: lassitude, distention of the abdomen, diarrhea, greasy tongue coating, and soft pulse. Jaundice is often a sign of dampness. If it is a local infection, dampness is usually manifested as exudation in the form of either mucous or purulent. Thus, from the traditional point of view, dysentery with bloody stools, pus and mucus, urinary infection with turbid urine, pelvic or vulvovaginal infection with profuse vaginal discharge are all attributed to damp-heat.

Herbal Therapies of Acute Infections

Herbal treatment of acute infections, aimed at elimination of the pathogens, has two main parts: one for the disease and the other for the syndrome. It is difficult to make a distinction between the two, however, for the syndrome diagnosis often includes the cause of disease. Only in a few exceptions is there a specific herbal treatment for the disease. For example, Radix Dichroae (dichora root) or Herba Artemisiae (sweet wormwood) for malaria. Since most acute infections are caused by pathogens of "toxic heat," "heat-clearing and detoxifying" drugs are indicated; administration of these herbs can be taken as causal

---

* Cornu Rhinoceri was used in the past, but nowadays it is replaced by Cornu Bubali (buffalo horn) because the use of the former is banned for the protection of rare wild animals.

therapy. Commonly used herbs in this category are: Flos Lonicerae (honeysuckle flower), Fructus Forsythiae (forsythia fruit), Radix Isatidis (dyer's woad root), Herba Taraxaci (dandelion herb), Herba Houttuyniae (houttuynia), Herba Andrographitis (green chiretta), Radix Scutellariae (scutellaria root), Rhizoma Coptidis (coptis root), Cortex Phellodendri (phellodendron bark) and Herba Violae (viola herb).

For infections caused by damp-heat, in which the principal treatment is to "clear the heat and eliminate damp," there are some similarities with the heat-clearing and detoxifying herbs. For example, Radix Scutellariae (scutellaria root), Rhizoma Coptidis (coptis root) and Cortex Phellodendri (phellodendron bark) are both "heat-clearing and damp-eliminating," and at the same time, "heat-clearing and detoxifying." There are also herbs which only work to clear heat and eliminate damp. Fructus Bruceae (brucea fruit), which is used orally for amebic dysentery and topically for trichomonal vaginitis; Radix Pulsatillae (pulsatilla root), which is used orally for bacillary dysentery and externally for trichomonas vaginitis; and Herba Artemisiae Scopariae (oriental wormwood), which is used for icteric hepatitis.

Ordinarily, the prescription is a combination of ingredients for relieving the syndrome and treating the disease. For example, the formula *Yin Qiao San* (Powder of Lonicera and Forsythia), which is customarily used for treating respiratory infections at the early stage with exterior syndrome, consists of the following ingredients: Flos Lonicerae (honeysuckle flower), Fructus Forsythiae (forsythia fruit), Fructus Arctii (artium fruit), Herba Menthae (peppermint), Herba Schizonepetae (schizonepeta), Semen Sojae Praeparatum (prepared soybean), Radix Platycodi (platycodon root), Rhizoma Phragmitis (reed rhizome), Radix Glycyrrhizae (licorice) and Herba Lophatheri (lophatherum).

In this formula, Herba Schizonepetae and Semen Sojae Praeparatum are diaphoretics for relieving the exterior syndrome; Fructus Arctii and Herba Menthae also help to relieve the exterior syndrome and expel heat from the exterior portion of the body. Flos Lonicerae and Fructus Forsythiae are heat-clearing and detoxifying herbs chiefly used against the pathogens. Radix Platycodi and Radix Glycyrrhizae are used for relieving sore throat and cough. Herba Lophatheri and Rhizoma Phragmitis are also heat-clearing herbs, the latter particularly good for the heat in the lung.

From the above analysis, it can be seen that traditional treatment of infections is by no means just symptomatic. Comparing the above formula with *Qing Ying Tang* (Decoction for Clearing Heat from the *Ying* System), which is indicated in infections with interior syndrome Pattern II, the rationality of herbal treatment becomes even more evident.

Qing Ying Tang is composed of the following ingredients: Cornu Rhinoceri (rhinoceros horn), Radix Rehmanniae (rehmannia root), Radix Scrophulariae (scrophularia root), Radix Ophiopogonis (ophiopogon root), Radix Salviae Miltiorrhizae (red sage root), Flos Lonicerae (honeysuckle flower), Fructus Forsythiae (forsythia fruit), Herba Lophatheri (lophatherum) and Rhizoma Coptidis (coptis root).

Among these ingredients, Cornu Rhinoceri and Radix Rehmanniae are used for clearing heat from the *ying* system; Flos Lonicerae, Fructus Forsythiae and Radix Coptidis are heat-clearing and detoxifying herbs. As exuberant heat is apt to impair body fluid, Radix Scrophulariae and Radix Ophiopogonis are added to promote its production and clear the heat. Herba Lophatheri and Radix Salviae Miltiorrhizae are added to strengthen the action of clearing heat from the *ying* system.

Comparison of the two formulas shows that the latter acts more powerfully against toxic heat, and the routes of expelling heat are different. In the former, the pathogen is expelled through diaphoresis from the exterior portion of the body, while in the latter, the pathogen is expelled from the *ying* system. In addition, since the condition is much more serious when toxic heat has entered the *ying* system, causing disturbance of the heart (central nervous system) and impairment of body fluid, ingredients such as Cornu Rhinoceri for treating impaired consciousness and others for promoting production of body fluid are added.

It's not difficult to comprehend the different routes to expel heat at different stages of an infectious disease or in different infectious diseases, even from a modern medical perspective. For example, in an upper respiratory infection at the early stage manifested as an exterior syndrome, treatment with diaphoretic antipyretics and ingredients to counteract the invading pathogen appears quite reasonable. In a severe case of infection with high fever and impaired consciousness, the Qing Ying Tang formula is obviously the right treatment. Modern pharmacological studies have given further evidence to show the rationale of the above-mentioned herbal treatment.

Pharmacological Studies of the Herbal Therapies
I. Herbs for Relieving Syndromes

The diaphoretic and antipyretic effects of herbs used for expelling heat in the exterior syndrome have been confirmed by clinical observation. Modern pharmacological studies have demonstrated the antipyretic effect of Herba Schizonepetae (schizonepeta) and Folium Mori (mulberry leaf) in inducing sweating. Radix Ledebouriellae (ledebouriella root) relieves fever in viral respiratory infections, probably due to its antiviral action, and Flos Chrysanthemi (chrysanthemum flower), due to its antibacterial action.

Of the herbs used for half-exterior half-interior syndromes, Radix Bupleuri (bupleurum root) is a potent antipyretic. It has been shown to reduce normal body temperature in animals. Pharmacological studies have also revealed its antiviral, antibacterial and anti-inflammatory effects. Radix Scutellariae (scutellaria root) is a heat-clearing and detoxifying herb whose pharmacological actions will be discussed later.

Among the herbs that treat interior syndromes, Gypsum Fibrosum (gypsum) has attracted much interest. It is very effective for relieving high fever in the syndrome involving the *qi* system of pattern I-a, for example in epidemic encephalitis B, which is refractory to even West antipyretics. The antipyretic effect of gypsum has also been demonstrated in animal experiments, not through induction of sweating, however, but rather through inhibition of the heat-regulatory center. It should be noted that only uncalcined gypsum works as such; once calcined, its antipyretic action is utterly lost, and it can only be used as plaster. The active component for relieving fever, therefore, is some other substance than the calcium sulfate in uncalcined gypsum.

Rhizoma Anemarrhenae (anemarrhena rhizome) has been demonstrated to have an antipyretic effect and exercise some inhibitory action on bacteria.

Radix et Rhizoma Rhei (rhubarb) for pattern I-b is a drug worthy of special attention; its pharmacological use will be discussed later in this chapter. Although used as a cathartic in Western medicine, its application in traditional Chinese medicine goes far beyond the treatment of constipation. Because of its potent effect on many acute conditions, it is called "the chief of drugs."

Calculus Bovis (ox gallstone) has been shown to inhibit the central nervous system in experimental studies, thus its effect on restless, delirium or convulsion due to high fever.

Cornu Rhinoceri (rhinoceros horn) is both an antipyretic and a good cardiotonic, as shown in modern experimental studies. radix rehmanniae (rehmannia root) is an antibacterial agent, which works particularly to neutralize bacterial endotoxins.

From the above, we can see that traditional treatment of various syndromes in infectious diseases has not only proven effective through hundreds of years of practice, but is now gaining recognition in modern scientific research.

II. Heat-clearing and Detoxifying Therapies

Heat-clearing and detoxifying herbs have been extensively studied for causal treatment of acute infections. Although discovered empirically, modern studies of these herbs have shown their multiple beneficial actions on infections.

1. Antiviral and Antibacterial Actions

Experimental studies have revealed that many heat-clearing and detoxifying herbs have antiviral actions. For example, Flos Lonicerae, Fructus Forsythiae, Folium Isatidis (dyer's woad leaf), Radix Isatidis (dyer's woad root), Herba Houttuyniae, Radix Scutellariae (scutellaria root), and Cortex Phellodendri (phellodendron bark) have an inhibitory action on Asian influenza virus A; Flos Lonicerae and Rhizoma Belamcandae (blackberrylily rhizome) inhibit ECHO virus; Cortex Phellodendri and Rhizoma Polygoni Cuspidati (giant knotweed rhizome) have an effect on hepatitis B antigen; and Herba Taraxaci, Herba Houttuyniae and Herba Andrographitis (green chiretta) can retard the cellular changes caused by viruses.

Most heat-clearing and detoxifying herbs have been found to have antibacterial actions of varying degree and range. Flos Lonicerae (honeysuckle flower), Fructus Forsythiae (forsythia fruit), Herba Taraxaci (dandelion herb), Herba Violae (viola herb), Rhizoma Coptidis (coptis root) and Herba Houttuyniae (houttuynia) have an inhibitory action on Gram positive bacteria (such as staphylococcus, streptococcus, pneumococcus and diphtheria bacillus) and Gram negative bacteria (such as typhoid and paratyphoid bacilli, dysentery bacillus and colibacillus).

It should be noted that the above data for bacteriostasis obtained in vitro cannot explain all the clinical results. Except for a few heat-clearing and detoxifying herbs such as Herba Houttuyniae (houttuynia) and Rhizoma Coptidis (coptis root), many of the herbs in this group, though bacteriostatic, are not as potent as antibiotics, and their effective blood level can hardly be achieved in clinical treatment with an ordinary oral dosage. But clinically, the results of herbal treatment of many bacterial infections are quite satisfactory. For example, a study of 191 patients with respiratory infections and high fever treated with heat-clearing and detoxifying herbs showed that in 67.85% body temperature was returned to normal in three days, and 93% were cured in one to two weeks. The results were comparable with antibiotic treatment. This high effectiveness rate can partly be explained by the combination of heat-clearing and detoxifying herbs which may lend a synergic action, but other therapeutic functions besides direct antimicrobial action may play an even more important role.

Tissue damage and complications in acute infections are not actually caused by the bacteria, but rather by the toxins. Except polymyxin B, most antibiotics have nothing to do with bacterial endotoxins. Investigation of heat-clearing and detoxifying herbs, however, has shown that many act to degrade endotoxins, enhance the function of mononuclear macrophages, and strengthen the lysosomes; in a word, they counteract the bacterial endotoxins. Further studies have shown their range of pharmacological actions which play a part in the treatment of infections. The main actions of commonly used heat-clearing and detoxifying herbs are summarized in Table III-1.

2. Detoxifying Action

It has been found that many heat-clearing and detoxifying herbs can counteract bacterial endotoxins. Radix Coptidis (coptis root) and Cortex Moutan Radicis (moutan bark) attenuate the toxicity of Staphylococcus aureus by inhibiting coagulase formation even at the concentration when no antibacterial action can be demonstrated. Tissue injury by Staphylococcus aureus is thus remarkably ameliorated.

Detoxication by other heat-clearing and detoxifying herbs has been carried out on animals in Nankai Hospital, Tianjin. In rabbits inoculated with typhoid endotoxin, an administration of Flos Lonicerae (honeysuckle flower), Fructus Forsythiae (forsythia fruit), Herba Taraxaci (dandelion herb) or Herba Violae (viola herb) relieved the fever, restored the reduced white blood cell count, and prolonged survival of the animals.

Since severe complications of acute infections are caused by the toxins released by bacteria, and most antibiotics in Western medicine have no effect on toxins or increase the release of endotoxins by de-

Table III-1
Main Pharmacological Actions of Commonly used Heat-clearing and Detoxifying Herbs

	Anti-bacterial	Anti-viral	Anti-inflammatory	Anti-pyretic	Detoxifying	Immune-enhancing	Other actions
Flos Lonicerae	+	+	+	+	+	+	diuretic
Fructus Forsythiae	+	+	+	+	+	+	cardiotonic diuretic liver-protecting
Folium Isatidis	+	+	+	+		+	
Radix Isatidis	+	+	+	+		+	
Herba Taraxaci	+				+		diuretic cholagogic liver-protecting
Herba Violae	+		+		+		
Herba Houttuyniae	+	+	+	+		+	
Herba Andrographitis	+	+				+	
Rhizoma Coptidis	+	+		+	+	+	antiprozoal sedative
Radix Scutellariae	+	+		+		+	diuretic sedative antiallergic hypotensive
Cortex Phellodendri	+	+	+				diuretic

stroying the bacteria, a new idea was naturally evoked: use antibiotics in combination with heat-clearing and detoxifying herbs to treat severe bacterial infections (particularly septicemia with complications). Undertaken by Tianjin Institute of Emergency Medicine, combined treatment has raised the cure rate of severe cases of septicemia complicated with toxic shock to 89% (which is 20% higher than the cure rate of similar cases treated with Western medicine alone).

3. Anti-inflammatory Action

Inflammation is the chief pathological change with infections. It has been demonstrated that many heat-clearing and detoxifying herbs act on various links of the inflammatory process. For instance, Fructus Forsythiae (forsythia fruit) inhibits inflammatory exudation; Radix Coptidis (coptis root) accelerates the subsidence of inflammation; and

Radix Scutellariae (scutellaria root) counteracts inflammation caused by allergic reaction. The therapeutic effect of these herbs are thus also associated with their anti-inflammatory actions.

4. Antipyretic Action

Some heat-clearing and detoxifying herbs have been demonstrated to have marked antipyretic effect in animal experiments. It is interesting to note that as they reduce fever without inducing much sweating, their antipyretic mechanism differs from that of antipyretic herbs which reduce fever chiefly through diaphoresis.

5. Actions on Host Immune Function

Medicinal herbs of this category act extensively on the human immune function. Rhizoma Coptidis (coptis root), Radix Scutellariae (scutellaria root) and Herba Andrographitis (green chiretta) enhance phagocytosis of leukocytes and reticulo-endothelial cells; Herba Houttuyniae (houttuynia) raises non-specific immunity by increasing the properdin level; Herba Taraxaci (dandelion herb), Rhizoma Coptidis (coptis root) and Radix Scutellariae (scutellaria root) elevate the lymphocyte transformation rate; and Radix Scutellariae (scutellaria root) and Rhizoma Coptidis (coptis root) inhibit allergic reaction.

6. Other Actions

This final category of herbs works in other ways to treat infections, as a diuretic for urinary infections, or as a cholagogic for biliary infections. These actions also extend the use of heat-clearing and detoxifying herbs to diseases other than infections.

III. Use of Rhubarb in Acute Infections

Treatment of interior syndrome pattern I-a with rhubarb is worth special mention. Rhubarb is a well-known cathartic both in Western medicine and traditional Chinese medicine, but its use in the treatment of infections is particular to the latter. Clinical studies have confirmed that it is effective for various infections such as erysipelas, acute mastitis, appendicitis and bacillary dysentery, but it is particularly effective when an infectious disease is accompanied by syndrome pattern I-b as described above. It is also useful in the prevention and early treatment of acute respiratory distress syndrome, a serious complication that may be encountered in acute infections. Experimental studies have revealed that rhubarb inhibits a variety of bacteria to various degrees; it is most potent against staphylococcus and streptococcus, but also works against typhoid and paratyphoid bacilli, dysentery bacillus and diphtheria bacillus. The active components of rhubarb are rhein, emodin, and aloe-emodin, which inhibit oxidation and dehydrogenation in glycometabolism of the bacteria as well as synthesis of protein and nucleic acid. The concentration of rhein, emodin or aloe-emodin required for bacteriostasis is less than 100 $\mu g/ml$.

Besides bacteria, many species of fungi, influenza virus, Amoeba dysenteriae and Trichomonas vaginalis are inhibited by rhubarb.

The chief therapeutic action of rhubarb in treatment of acute infections may not depend solely on its bacteria-inhibiting effect. In acute bacterial infections of the intestines (such as acute bacillary dysentery), there is accumulation of bacteria and toxins released by the bacteria in the intestines which cause pathological changes and clinical symptoms. Rhubarb can empty the bowels of the accumulated contents (including bacteria and their toxin), reducing the production of endotoxin in the bowels, and help the excretion of endotoxin through the bowels. In other infections, even if the primary lesion is not in the intestinal tract, putrefactive fermentation may occur there due to high fever, electrolyte disturbance or microbial toxins which inhibit intestinal secretion and motility, thus producing toxic substances. This aggravates the disease and brings about the clinical manifestations as described in syndrome pattern I-b. Use of rhubarb to expel these toxic substances makes sense. Other cathartics such as mirabilite (sodium sulfate) may be used, though rhubarb works best.

It is interesting to note that recent research has found rhubarb an effective agent against platelet aggregation, arteriolar contraction and bronchial spasm, particularly in cases of acute infection. All of these pathological changes are risky factors in a severe infection, as increased platelet aggregation may lead to disseminated intravascular coagulation, arteriolar contraction to toxic shock, and bronchial spasm to respiratory distress syndrome, any of which can lead to death.

Since rhubarb has so many therapeutic effects, it is widely used in the treatment of infections and other diseases. A controlled study by Beijing Friendship Hospital has shown that treating acute pneumonia with rhubarb and heat-clearing and detoxifying herbs is superior to antibiotics for relief of fever and inflammation.

Traditional Treatment of Chronic Infections

From the viewpoint of traditional Chinese medicine, in chronic infections the key point is deficiency of body resistance rather than invasion of pathogens. In treatment, therefore, emphasis is usually put on strengthening body resistance through administration of tonics. Elimination therapy may also be indicated, but the route of elimination is often different from those mentioned for acute infections; diaphoretics and cathartics in particular should be avoided because they further impair body resistance.

Examples of Herbal Treatment for Infectious Diseases

I. Influenza

Influenza is an acute respiratory infection, virus-induced, which is characterized by the abrupt onset of systemic symptoms: chill, fever, headache, myalgia and malaise, and accompanied by respiratory tract signs, particularly cough and sore throat. Outbreaks usually occur in winter or early spring. Influenza was thus traditionally believed to fit in the category of "epidemic febrile disease caused by wind" or "epidemic spring fever" and has been treated successfully with herbal medicine.

In a diagnosis of syndromes, most influenza patients exhibit exterior syndrome (attack of the exterior by wind-heat) at the early stage, and in syndrome pattern I-a with the *lung* involved (heat in the *lung*) soon thereafter. The point of differentiation between the two is in the chilliness: In exterior syndrome, there is chilliness though body temperature has not reached its extreme; in "heat in the *lung*" syndrome there is a high fever but no more chilliness.

Treatment of influenza comprises two principal parts: treatment of the disease and treatment of the syndrome. As an epidemic febrile disease, its causal pathogen is believed to be "toxic heat." Heat-clearing and detoxifying herbs are therefore employed. These commonly used have already been mentioned in the previous section, such as Flos Lonicerae (honeysuckle flower), Fructus Forsythiae (forsythia fruit) and Radix Isatidis (isatis root, also called dyer's woad root). The first two are used in the formula *Yin Qiao San* (Powder of Lonicera and Forsythia). Effective against influenza and other respiratory infections at the early stage, ready-to-use preparations (pills and tablets) of this formula are widely used in China. Radix Isatidis alone acts potently against the influenza viruses and has been made into a dosage form of granules. As there are no other ingredients for treating the syndromes, it is used for mild cases and to prevent outbreaks of the illness.

So far as the syndromes are concerned, diaphoretic antipyretics such as Herba Schizonepetae and Radix Bupleuri are employed for relieving exterior syndrome, and non-diaphoretic antipyretics such as Gypsum Fibrosum and Rhizoma Anemarrhenae are administered for interior syndrome of heat in the *lung*.

A clinical trial was carried out in our institute during an outbreak of influenza to evaluate the use of herbal therapies. Sixty-four patients were randomly divided into two groups: the first group was treated with only herbal medication, and the second (control group) with routine Western symptomatic drugs, such as aspirin for fever and antibiotics for prevention of secondary bacterial infections. The herbal therapies were of two types: the first, based on the *Yin Qiao San* formula, was administered to those with exterior syndrome; the second, without the diaphoretics, included a large dose of Gypsum Fibrosum and was administered to those with syndrome of heat in the *lung*. Before treatment, the two groups were comparable in terms of age, body temperature (38.6 ℃ on the average in both groups) and course of the disease. Body temperature of the patients treated with herbal medicines returned to normal in 1.3 days, while those in the control group receded in 2.4 days, the statistical difference being very significant ($P < 0.001$). It was noted in some cases that after taking aspirin, body temperature dropped sharply as a result of profuse sweating, but the symptoms returned after a few hours. Among those who received herbal treatment, none experienced profuse perspiration, and once the body temperature dropped, it did not rise again. It was also noted on follow-ups that the patients who received herbal treatment recovered faster and seldom complained of "postinfluenzal asthenia," a frequent complaint among patients in the control group, particularly those who had profuse sweating after taking aspirin.

II. Viral Hepatitis

Viral hepatitis is a systemic infection which primarily affects the liver. Among the five types (hepatitis A, hepatitis B, delta hepatitis, hepatitis C, and hepatitis E), hepatitis B occurs most commonly in China.

The earliest symptoms of acute viral hepatitis are nonspecific and variable. Anorexia, nausea and vomiting, fatigue, malaise, headache, cough and coryza may precede the onset of jaundice by one to two weeks. There may be low grade fever. Jaundice in acute hepatitis is usually diagnosed *yang* jaundice due to accumulation of damp-heat in the liver. Characterized by a lustrous yellow discoloration of the skin and sclera, it is accompanied by fever, bitter taste in the mouth, greasy tongue coating, and taut, slippery and rapid pulse. As an acute epidemic infectious disease, it is also considered the pathogenic agent. The principle of treatment is thus to eliminate dampness, clear up heat and remove toxins. Herbal therapy is usually bi-directional: to eliminate damp-heat and to clear up toxic heat. Among the herbs that eliminate damp-heat, Herba Artemisiae Scopariae (oriental wormwood), as recorded in *Shang Han Lun (Treatise on Febrile Diseases)* from the beginning of the 3rd century, in particular treats jaundice. Modern pharmacological research has revealed the advantageous effect of oriental wormwood on hepatitis. On the one hand, it promotes bile secretion, protects the liver from damage caused by chemicals, and enforces the detoxifying function of the liver; on the other hand, it inhibits the hepatitis virus. In addition, it has an antipyretic action and is an effective agent to reduce blood lipids to prevent atherosclerosis and fat deposit in the visceral organs (including the liver). Another important finding is that the low toxicity of oriental wormwood, making it safe for patients with a diseased liver.

Radix et Rhizoma Rhei (rhubarb) is often used in combination with oriental wormwood. The pharmacological actions of rhubarb have already been discussed. An additional benefit is the heightened cholagogic effect of oriental wormwood when taken with rhubarb.

Heat-clearing and detoxifying herbs commonly used in the treatment of acute hepatitis are Radix Isatidis (dyer's woad root) and Radix Scutellariae (scutellaria root). Their action against hepatitis viruses in experimental studies provides a modern explanation of the traditional treatment.

Since most patients with acute hepatitis can recover spontaneously, herbal treatment, though effective, is not so spectacular as with chronic hepatitis. In Western medicine, glucocorticoid therapy is recommended for treatment of chronic hepatitis, but its side effects are difficult to avoid. Alpha interferon has shown some promise in reducing or eliminating viral replication in chronic active hepatitis, but it cannot be recommended for general use at present. Treating chronic hepatitis thus remains a difficult problem.

In recent decades, extensive studies have been carried out on the traditional treatment of chronic hepatitis. Encouraging results have been repeatedly reported by physicians from different institutions, who prescribed compound decoctions according to traditional differential diagnosis of syndromes. The therapeutic modalities were so complicated that even a brief description is beyond the scope of this book. However, based upon these experiences, individual herbs have been studied. A few of the more interesting ones are listed below:

1. Fructus Schisandrae (Schisandra Fruit) and Diphenyldiester

In the traditional treatment of chronic hepatitis, schisandra fruit is particularly effective for lowering the serum aminotransferase level. Diphenyldiester is a substance extracted from schisandra fruit. An immediate drop in the serum aminotransferase level was found in 90% of the cases treated with this agent. Aggravation of the patient's condition was nonetheless reported in a few cases during the course of diphenyldiester therapy.

2. Polyporus Umbellatus (Umbellate Pore-fungus) and Its Polysaccharide

The use of umbellate pore-fungus in the treatment of jaundice was also introduced in *Shang Han Lun* (*Treatise on Febrile Disease*). Used in combination with sweet wormwood, it is indicated in cases of jaundice when skin discoloration is dull, there is no distinctive fever, but digestive symptoms such as anorexia, stomach distress and loose stools are predominant.

Based on its clinical effect, a polysaccharide of this pore-fungus was extracted by the Institute of Materia Medica, China Academy of Traditional Chinese Medicine. Experimental studies revealed that Polyporus Umbellatus Polysaccharide (PUP) acts to enhance immunity. Randomly controlled clinical trials of 319 cases of chronic hepatitis carried out in nine hospitals in 1981 showed encouraging results: The effective rates of reducing the serum aminotransferase level and eliminating viral replication in the PUP group were much higher than those of the control groups. Since the drugs used in the control groups varied by hospital, another double-blind pairing trial was performed on 80 cases in 1985. Forty mg of PUP was administered intramuscularly every day for three months, with a 10-day interval each month. A placebo of highly diluted Radix Salviae Miltiorrhizae solution was administered to the control group under the same scheme as the PUP injection. The diagnosis was established by liver biopsy in all 80 cases. Patients' age, duration of the disease, serum aminotransferase level and virus indices were approximately the same in the two groups. By the end of the treatment, in the PUP group 91% showed clinical improvement, 58.3% had a marked drop in the serum aminotransferase level, and 62.4% experienced reduction or total elimination of HBsAg titer, while in the control group, these figures were 42%, 34.5% and 31.3% respectively. So far as HBeAg is concerned, it was changed to negative in 10 of the 12 positive cases of the PUP group, but only two of the 11 positive cases of the control group showed such an effect. The above results showed some promise in reducing or eliminating virus replication.

Experimental studies in animals also showed that PUP acts to increase storage of glycogen in the liver, mitigates liver damage caused by various toxic chemicals, and stimulates regeneration of liver cells. All these data suggest the beneficial effect of PUP in the treatment of liver damage caused by viruses.

III. Malaria

Malaria is one of the most widely spread communicable diseases; it is particularly common in the tropics and subtropics but also occurs in some temperate regions. It is an acute, often severe, and sometimes protracted disease caused by parasitic protozoa of the genus Plasmodium. There are generally three stages: cold stage (shivering chill), hot stage (high fever) and sweating stage (defervescence). Since alternate spells of bedshaking chills followed by high fever are so remarkable, this disease was recognized by the Chinese thousands of years ago and named *nue* (瘧) in *Canon of Medicine*. This term is still used for malaria in the Chinese language.

"Malaria" was originally an Italian word which means bad air. In traditional Chinese medicine the cause of malaria, particularly in epidemic regions, was believed to be *zhangqi*, which also means bad or evil air. In China dozens of herbs were found to be antimalarial. Quinine, the alkaloid found in the bark of the South American cinchona tree, was the most well-known drug for malaria in other parts of the world in the past. The use of cinchona bark for the treatment of malarial fevers dates back to the 17th century. For 300 years, until the Japanese occupation of Javanese cinchona plantations, this powdered bark was the only effective remedy for malaria in many countries. Although quinine can now be manufactured, it is still extracted from cinchona bark. This is one example of medicinal herbs in the development of therapeutics.

From 1946 to 1966 chloroquine was used widely to treat malaria. Unfortunately, chloroquine-resistant malaria has prevailed in many areas since that time. Though new antimalarial drugs have been synthesized for chloroquine-resistant strains of plasmodium, they are constantly challenged by the development of new strains of the disease. Treatment of cerebral malaria has also been a problem; the mortality rate is about 20%. Chinese researchers have thus gone on to develop new antimalarial drugs from traditional herbs.

Among the antimalarial herbs recorded in traditional Chinese medical literature, Herba Artemisiae Chinghao (*qinghao* or sweet wormwood) is often noted. It consists of the dried aerial parts of Artemisia annua L. (family Compositae) which grows in abundance all over China. The herb was first recorded as an antimalarial in *Zhou Hou Bei Ji Fang (A Handbook of Prescriptions for Emergencies)* written by Ge Hong in 340 A.D. Li Shizhen also stated in his famous *Ben Cao Gang Mu (Compendium of Materia Medica)* in 1596 A.D. that chill and fever caused by malaria can be relieved by compound *qinghao* preparations of Herba Artemisiae Chinghao.

In the late 1960s, clinical studies were performed on the use of Herba Artemisiae Chinghao as an antimalarial, but its therapeutic effect was neither pronounced nor consistent. An active antimalarial fraction of Artemisia annua L. was then isolated in 1971, from which a new antimalarial was isolated the following year and named Qinghaosu (Artemisine). Clinical trials on chloroquine-resistant malaria revealed satisfactory results with the artemisine. In a series of 65 chloroquine-resistant cases artemisine cured all of them clinically; the relapse rate after four weeks was 7.7%, much lower than that with quinine therapy. In non-chloroquine-resistant malaria, artemisine works better than chloroquine. In an epidemic area in Southwest China, 60 cases of pernicious malaria were all cured with artemisine, while among the 80 cases treated with chloroquine, only 76 (95%) were cured. Artemisine works faster than chloroquine: in the above pernicious cases, Plasmodium falciparum disappeared from the blood in an average of 37 hours when artemisine tablets were administered and in 29.7 hours when oil suspension of artemisine was used, but it took an average of 65.7 hours in chloroquine therapy. Toxic and side effects of artemisine are mild. The only disadvantage to this drug in the treatment of pernicious malaria is the high incidence of relapse, particularly when the drug is administered orally. Intramuscular injection of its oil solution or oil suspension has greatly reduced the relapse rate. A few new compounds such as artemetherin and sodium artesunate have been derived from artemisine to further improve its therapeutic effect.

CHAPTER IV
USE OF TONICS IN TRADITIONAL CHINESE MEDICINE

Chinese herbal medication has many distinctive features, one of which is the wide use of tonics. The term "tonic" was also used in Western medicine in the past; it was a class of medicinal preparations believed to have the power to restore normal tone to tissues (e.g., bitter tonic— used to stimulate the appetite and improve digestion, such as gentian; cardiac tonic— used to strengthen cardiac action, such as digitalis; hematic tonic— used to improve the quality of the blood, such as iron; neurotonic— used to improve the tone of the nervous system).

In traditional Chinese medicine, the word "tonic" has a much broader meaning and refers to various medicines which treat "deficiency syndromes." "Deficiency syndrome" in traditional Chinese medicine is different from "deficiency disease" in Western medicine. The latter is defined as disease due to the lack of some element in the diet, but the former includes numerous diseases characterized by deficiency of vital capacity, including insufficient body resistance, diminished function, reduced metabolism, consumption of tissue or lack of essential substances in the body.

Deficiency Syndromes

Traditional Chinese medicine attaches great importance to deficiency syndromes or conditions, because disease is seen as a process of struggle between the vital capacity of the human body (particularly body resistance or genuine *qi*) and pathogenic factors. The occurrence and development of disease is either due to deficiency of the vital capacity, excess of pathogenic factors, or both.

Generally speaking, vital capacity consists of two main aspects: *yin* and *yang*. *Yin* and *yang* are terms from ancient Chinese philosophy which refer to two opposite aspects of matters in the universe interrelated with each other. As medical terms, they represent the two principal aspects of the human body. *Yin* refers to the structure and substances essential for maintaining normal functional activities such as vital essence, blood, body fluids and nutrients. *Yang* refers to the functional aspect of the human body, including functional activities and metabolism, as well as the required heat energy and dynamic energy for these processes.

Deficiency syndromes can be divided into two main categories: deficiency of *yin* and deficiency of *yang*. In clinical practice, it is customary to separate deficiency of blood from deficiency of *yin* and deficiency of *qi* (vital energy, i.e., dynamic energy for physiological processes) from deficiency of *yang*. Therefore, there are four types of deficiency syndromes: deficiency of blood, deficiency of *yin*, deficiency of *qi* and deficiency of *yang*. There are also complicated cases of deficiency syndromes, such as deficiency of both *qi* and blood, deficiency of both *qi* and *yin*, deficiency of both *yin* and *yang*.

The common clinical manifestations of deficiency of blood are: pallor, pale tongue and lips, and scanty menses for women.

The common clinical manifestations of deficiency of *yin* are: dryness in the mouth, constipation, reddened tongue with scanty coating, and thready pulse. Secondary symptoms are: insomnia and dream-disturbed sleep with deficiency of the *heart yin*, dryness of the eyes, blurred vision, dizziness and tinnitus when the *liver yin* is impaired, dry cough, hoarseness, and night sweating when the *lung yin* is insufficient, weakness of the loins and knees, sterility or infertility with deficiency of the *kidney yin*.

The common clinical manifestations of deficiency of *qi* are: weakness, lassitude, spontaneous sweating and weak pulse. There are also diminished functional processes of corresponding visceral organs, such as cardiac palpitation and shortness of breath when the *heart qi* is impaired; cough, dyspnea or liability to repeated colds when the *lung qi* is insufficient; anorexia, abdominal distention, loose stools or edema when the *spleen qi* is weakened; lumbago, weakness of the legs, impotence, hyposexuality, or oliguria and edema when the *kidney qi* is impaired.

Deficiency of *yang* is often much like deficiency of *qi*, but with cold manifestations such as cold limbs, and aversion to cold, either general or local.

From the above, it can be seen that deficiency syndromes may occur in numerous diseases and involve many kinds of chronic ailments, especially if there is no acute exacerbation. Even acute disease may show deficiency syndromes in the late or convalescent stage.

Classification of Tonics

Tonics are classified in accordance with the deficiency syndromes they treat. Generally speaking, there are four groups: drugs for nourishing blood (blood tonics), drugs for replenishing *yin* (*yin* tonics), drugs for tonifying *qi* (*qi* tonics) and drugs for reinforcing *yang* (*yang* tonics). They can be further classified according to the visceral organ which the tonic acts on: some *yin* tonics are particularly effective for replenishing the *lung yin* and some for replenishing the *kidney yin*; some *qi* tonics are particularly effective for tonifying the *spleen qi*, and some for tonifying the *lung qi*.

The representative tonics of each group and their actions are listed as follows:

1. *Qi* Tonics — medicines which invigorate *qi* (dynamic energy for various physiological activities, including resistance against disease) indicated in the treatment of *qi* deficiency.

Radix Ginseng (ginseng): In China, ginseng refers to the dried root of Panax ginseng C. A. Mey, and is often called Jilin ginseng for the product from the mountainous areas in Jilin Province. This well-known tonic works primarily to replenish *qi* in cases of prostration or shock (particularly cardiogenic shock). It can also be used as a roborant to build up health in cases of debility or chronic disease and to treat frigidity in females and impotence in males. Its cardiotonic function has recently been demonstrated in the treatment of heart failure.

The dried root of Panax ginseng C. A. Mey is not the same as American ginseng, which is the dried root of Panax quinquefolium. The latter has less potent action to replenish *qi* but is more effective for promoting production of body fluids; it is used widely for debility accompanied by impairment of body fluid, as with patients after febrile diseases who suffer general weakness and dryness. Both Jilin ginseng and American ginseng are better taken individually without other ingredients. The usual daily dose is 3-9g in a decoction. It should be emphasized that Radix Ginseng is only indicated for those with deficiency syndromes. If taken by a healthy person, particularly one with a strong constitution, it may cause adverse effects such as epistaxis, ulceration in the mouth or hypertension.

Radix Astragali (astragalus root): The Chinese name for Radix Astragali is *huangqi* (黄耆), in which *huang* (黄) means yellow and *qi* (耆), a respected old person in the community, indicating its status among all medicinal herbs.

Its main action is to replenish *qi* and strengthen superficial resistance against general weakness, particularly for those suffering from *qi* deficiency with spontaneous sweating and vulnerability to repeated respiratory infections, chronic diarrhea, massive uterine bleeding or anemia. It is also used in surgery to promote discharge of pus, regeneration of tissues and healing of ulcers. Recent clinical trials have shown its use in treating chronic nephritis with albuminuria and diabetes mellitus. The daily dose varies from 10 to 30g.

Radix Acanthopanacis Senticosi (acanthopanax root): This is a *qi*-replenishing drug that also acts as a tranquilizer to treat general weakness accompanied by insomnia. The daily dose is 10-30g.

II. Blood Tonics— medicines that enrich the blood, indicated in treatment of blood deficiency.

Radix Angelicae Sinensis (Chinese angelica root): This is the most important medicinal herb used in gynecology, particularly for treating menstrual disorders. Its Chinese name is *danggui* (当归), of which *dang* (当) means to be obliged, and *gui* (归) means "return." The name came from a story about a woman who suffered from a severe menstrual disorder and whose husband left her for this reason. After taking Radix Angelicae Sinensis, her normal menstruation was restored, and he was obliged to return home.

This blood tonic not only promotes blood regeneration and blood circulation but also regulates menstruation and works as an analgesic. Its first indication is for menstrual disorders, including dysmenorrhea. Used in combination with Radix Astragali, it is prescribed for treatment of anemia, and alone to treat rheumatoid arthritis and various traumata, as it promotes local blood circulation and helps relieve pain. Besides these tonic actions, it may cause mild laxation and is therefore indicated for those with blood deficiency complicated by constipation. Daily dosage is 6-10g.

Radix Rehmanniae Praeparata (prepared rehmannia root): Fresh rehmannia root is a herbal drug for clearing heat and promoting secretion of body fluids. It is used to treat various conditions of *yin* deficiency with heat manifestations, such as diabetes mellitus. After being steamed, the prepared root works to replenish blood and vital essence as well as body fluids. It is frequently used to treat anemia and other conditions such as lumbago, noctural emission and menstrual disorders due to deficiency of *yin* and blood. The daily dosage is 10-15g.

Colla Corii Asini (ass-hide gelatin): This glue prepared from the skin of ass is used to nourish the blood and stop bleeding when there is deficiency of blood and various kinds of bleeding. It is indicated particularly in consumptive diseases with anemia, general weakness, insomnia, dry cough or hemoptysis. It is also frequently used for treating excessive menstrual discharge and possible miscarriage. Daily dosage is 3-10g, after being melted in hot water.

III. *Yin* Tonics— medicines that replenish *yin* (structural substances, vital essence, body fluids, nutrients and other substances essential for resistance against disease and normal physical and visceral functioning), indicated in the treatment of *yin* deficiency.

Radix Ophiopogonis (ophiopogon root): This acts to replenish vital essence and promote secretion of body fluids, particularly secretion of the respiratory tract, and is often used to treat dry cough in consumptive diseases and diabetes mellitus manifested by thirstiness. An important drug for treating diphtheria, its antibacterial action has been recently demonstrated *in vitro*. In addition, it works as a cardio-tonic for treating palpitation. Daily dosage is 6-12g.

Fructus Lycii (wolfberry fruit): With the taste of grapes, this is often taken as a tonic in China, particularly by the aged. It works to replenish *yin* of the *liver* and *kidney*, and is therefore used to treat aching in the loins and knees, dizziness, tinnitus and blurred vision due to deficiency of *liver* and *kidney yin*. It is also used in the treatment of diabetes mellitus. Daily dosage is 6-12g.

Fructus Ligustri Lucidi (lucid ligustrum fruit): This is also a tonic for replenishing *yin* of the *liver* and *kidney*, and is used for weakness of the loins and knees, dizziness, tinnitus and blurred vision due to deficiency of *liver* and *kidney yin*. In addition, it can be used to prevent and treat premature graying. The daily dosage is 6-12g.

IV. *Yang* Tonics— medicines that invigorate *yang* (*qi* plus heat metabolism), indicated in the treatment of *yang* deficiency.

Cornu Cervi Pantotrichum (pilose deerhorn): This downy horn of a young male deer is used as a potent roborant to enhance strength, particularly in the *kidney* for treatment of intolerance to cold, loss of strength, impotence, spontaneous seminal emission and other symptoms of weakened vital function with chronic diseases. Daily dosage is 1-2g, pulverized and mixed with hot water.

Herba Epimedii (epimedium): This is a general roborant to promote strength and replenish the vital function of the *kidney*, especially in the sexual organs for treatment of sexual neurasthenia and climacteric syndrome. It is also effective for treating rheumatism.

Fructus Psoraleae (psoralea fruit): Acting to warm up the *kidney* and reinforce the vital function of sexual organs, it is used to treat impotence, nocturnal emission, and chronic diarrhea occurring daily just before dawn due to deficiency of *kidney yang*.

Modern Research on Tonics

According to the modern research on their pharmacological actions, tonics work in the following ways:

I. Action on Immune Functions (Table IV-1)

Most tonics enhance nonspecific immune functions; some work on specific immunity.

1. Nonspecific Immune Functions

(1) Increase of peripheral white blood cells. Both in animal experiments and in clinical practice, tonics such as Radix Ginseng (ginseng), Radix Codonopsis Pilosulae (pilose asiabell root), Rhizoma Atractylodis Macrocephalae (white atractylodes rhizome), Radix Astragali (astragalus root), Radix Rehmanniae (rehmannia root), Fructus Lycii (wolfberry fruit), Cornu Cervi Pantotrichum (pilose deerhorn), Ganoderma Lucidum (lucid ganoderma), Colla Corii Asini (ass-hide gelatin) increase peripheral white blood cells, particularly in cases of leukopenia.

(2) Increase of reticulo-endothelial phagocytosis. Many tonics, particularly *qi* tonics, increase the phagocytic function of the reticuloendothelial system in animal experiments.

(3) Astragalus root promotes the leukocyte production of interferon induced by the influenza virus.

2. Specific Immune Functions

(1) Many tonics such as Radix Ginseng (ginseng), Radix Astragali (astragalus root), and Fructus Schisandrae (schisandra fruit) increase the rate of lymphocyte transformation in healthy individuals.

(2) Radix Ginseng can elevate serum gamma-globulin and immunoglobulin-M levels. Radix Astragali can markedly increase the immunoglobulin-M level in healthy subjects. Radix Codonopsis Pilosulae, Rhizoma Atractylodis Macrocephalae and poria increase the serum immunoglobulin-G level. Fructus Lycii and Fructus Ligustri Lucidi increase humoral immunity.

Table IV-1

Action of Tonics on Immune Function

	Increasing phagocytosis of reticulo-endothelial cells	Increasing peripheral leukocytes	Enhancing cellular immunity	Enhancing humoral immunity
Qi Tonics				
Radix Ginseng	+	+	+	+
Radix Astragali	+	+	+	+
Radix Codonopsis Pilosulae	+	+	+	+
Blood Tonics				
Radix Angelicae Sinensis	+		+	
Colla Corii Asini		+	+	
Yin Tonics				
Radix Ophiopogonis	+	+		
Fructus Lycii	+	+	+	+
Fructus Ligustri Lucidi	+	+	+	+
Yang Tonics				
Cornu Cervi Pantotrichum		+		
Herba Epimedii	+	+	+	
Fructus Psoraleae		+	+	+

II. Action on Adaptability

Quite a few tonics help the body adapt to the external environment by resisting harmful stimuli and restoring disordered functions to normal through bi-directional regulation. For example, Radix Ginseng can restore the normal red blood cell count in polycythemia caused by cobalt nitrate, and increase the red blood cell count in hypocythemia caused by phenylhydrazine. This kind of bi-directional regulatory action is sometimes called the "adaptogen" effect. The Jade Screen Powder (cf. p.30), the principal ingredient Radix Astragali also has such an effect, as shown by the PFC test: It raises the immune response when it is low, and reduces it when it is high. Radix Rehmanniae, Radix Ophiopogonis and other *yin* tonics act to regulate the synthesis rate of nucleic acid, reducing it when it is high, and increasing it when it is low.

III. Action on the Endocrine System (Table IV-2)

Qi tonics and *yang* tonics exhibit the greatest effect on the endocrine system. Radix Ginseng stimulates pituitary secretion of ACTH and gonadotropic hormones, expediting sexual maturity in animals. Radix Acanthopanacis Senticosi also stimulates the adrenocortical and sexual glands. Radix Codonopsis Pilosulae can significantly elevate the plasma corticosterone level in mice. Herba Epimedii has a testosterone-like effect, and Fructus Psoraleae a weak estrogen-like effect.

IV. Action on Metabolism (Table IV-2)

Radix Ginseng has a regulatory effect on carbohydrate and lipid metabolism; it promotes biosynthesis of protein, DNA and RNA, and increases blood albumin and gamma-globulin substances. Radix Acanthopanacis Senticosi regulates blood sugar and promotes biosynthesis of nucleic acid and protein. Radix Astragali promotes metabolism of serum and liver protein.

Radix Angelicae Sinensis has been shown to protect animals in experiments from atherosclerosis; it also counteracts vitamin E deficiency. Radix Polygoni Multiflori reduces the blood cholesterol level and acts against atherosclerosis.

V. Action on the Cardiovascular System (Table IV-3)

Many tonics, particularly *qi* tonics, work on the cardiovascular system to increase myocardial contractive power, dilate blood vessels and reduce hypertension. Some are also effective for counteracting myocardial ischemia and arrhythmia. They are thus often used to treat heart failure, cardiogenic shock and coronary heart disease.

VI. Action on Hemopoiesis (Table IV-3)

Impaired hemopoiesis is manifested as anemia and leukopenia. According to traditional Chinese medicine, these diseases are usually diagnosed as deficiency of blood and deficiency of *qi*; in severe cases there is

Table IV-2

Action of Tonics on the Endocrine System and Metabolism

	Stimulation of adrenal cortex	Stimulation of sexual glands	Promotion of protein anabolism	Reduction of blood lipids	General roborant action
Qi Tonics					
Radix Ginseng	+	+	+	+	+
Radix Astragali			+		
Radix Codonopsis Pilosulae	+				
Blood Tonics					
Radix Angelicae Sinensis				+	
Colla Corii Asini					
Yin Tonics					
Radix Ophiopogonis	+				
Fructus Lycii				+	
Fructus Ligustri Lucidi					+
Yang Tonics					
Cornu Cervi Pantotrichum		+			+
Herba Epimedii		+		+	
Fructus Psoraleae		+			

also deficiency of *yang*. Clinical use of blood tonics, *qi* tonics and *yang* tonics has proven effective with these diseases. It has been shown in experiments that Radix Ginseng, Radix Codonopsis Pilosulae, Radix Astragali, Acanthopanacis Senticosi, Radix Angelicae Sinensis, Colla Corii Asini, and Cornu Cervi Pantotrichum promote hemopoiesis.

VII. Roborant Actions

Radix Ginseng improves mental and physical ability and alleviates fatigue. Cornu Cervi Pantotrichum increases working capability, improves sleeping and appetite, and reduces fatigue. In animal experiments, Rhizoma Atractylodis Macrocephalae and Fructus Ziziphi Jujubae have been shown to increase body weight and strength.

Indications of tonics:

Vital capacity is a general term referring to all the functions and substances required for maintaining health and protecting the body against disease. Since tonics act to restore or enhance various kinds of

Table IV-3

Action of Tonics on the Cardio-vascular System and Hemopoiesis

	Cardio-tonic action	Dilation of coronary artery	Dilation of cerebral vessels	Increase of RBC	Increase of Hb
Qi Tonics					
Radix Ginseng	+	+	+	+	+
Radix Astragali	+	+	+	+	+
Radix Codonopsis Pilosulae		+	+	+	+
Blood Tonics					
Radix Angelicae Sinensis		+		+	+
Colla Corii Asini				+	+
Yin Tonics					
Radix Ophiopogonis	+				
Fructus Lycii					
Fructus Ligustri Lucidi	+	+			
Yang Tonics					
Cornu Cervi Pantotrichum	+				
Herba Epimedii		+			
Fructus Psoraleae		+	+		

vital capacity, it is practically impossible to list all the indications. Those listed below are only a few examples.

Qi tonics: chronic gastrointestinal diseases (peptic ulcer, chronic gastritis, chronic colitis, chronic hepatitis, gastrointestinal neurosis, etc.), chronic respiratory diseases (chronic bronchitis, bronchial asthma in remission, etc.), *heart* diseases (*heart* failure, arrhythmias, etc.), and chronic nephritis.

Blood tonics: anemia, menstrual disorders with scanty menstrual flow.

Yin tonics: neurasthenia, hypertension, menopausal syndrome, chronic hepatitis, chronic gastritis, chronic nephritis, diabetes mellitus, sterility and infertility, pulmonary tuberculosis and other consumptive diseases.

Yang tonics: chronic gastrointestinal diseases characterized by aversion to cold, either general or local, adrenocortical insufficiency, hypothyroidism, chronic nephritis, and impotence.

These classifications are only suitable for the majority of cases of each disease. There are many exceptions. Most perplexing is that patients with one disease usually manifest several different syndrome patterns. This is true even when there is only a deficiency. For example, most cases of hypertension are diagnosed as deficiency of liver and kidney *yin* and can be treated with *yin* tonics; but there are also cases of deficiency of both *yin* and *yang*, in which *yin* and *yang* tonics should be used together. Furthermore, there are many overlaps, particularly with deficiency of *qi* and deficiency of *yang*, because *yang* deficiency can be formulated as *qi* deficiency plus manifestations of cold. Patients with chronic peptic ulcer usually suffer from epigastric pain (which can be alleviated by food) as well as from anorexia and lassitude, indicating a deficiency of *qi*. However, some peptic ulcer patients suffers from epigastric pain aggravated by exposure to cold and alleviated by warmth. In this case, *yang* deficiency of the stomach should be diagnosed and *yang* tonics administered. Combinations of two or more deficiency syndromes are not infrequently encountered; for example, deficiency of both *qi* and *yin*, or deficiency of both *qi* and blood. The following are some examples of tonic applications.

Tonic Treatment for Common Diseases

Chronic Bronchitis

Chronic bronchitis is a condition characterized by chronic or recurrent productive cough with profuse sputum. Its cause is not yet clear. Cigarette-smoking has been shown to be the most important predisposing factor. Some doctors of Western medicine hold that microorganisms infect the respiratory tract and cause this disease; others believe the infections are the result rather than the cause. Endogenous factor may also be involved. A genetic anomaly that affects mucus production may impair bronchial clearance, leading to recurrent or chronic infection. Bronchial allergens may increase secretion of mucus, making one more susceptible to bronchial infection. Exposure to cold that exacerbates the condition may also be related to constitutional hypersensitivity. No matter what the etiological factor, chronic bronchitis implies irreversible air obstruction; the main aims of treatment are to prevent further deterioration and treat secondary complications.

The traditional Chinese view on the etiology and pathogenesis of chronic bronchitis is quite different from that of modern Western medicine. Abnormal production of phlegm is taken as the main pathogenetic factor. In acute exacerbation invasion of the *lung* by heat brings about purulent phlegm which causes cough and even dyspnea. In chronic bronchitis without secondary infection, production of profuse nonpurulent phlegm is often attributed to impairment of the *spleen* function. In this case, the *lung* merely stores the phlegm until it is coughed up. Accumulation of phlegm in the *lung* renders it vulnerable to repeated attacks by exogenous pathogens, which may exacerbate the condition. In the later stages, there is shortness of breath and difficulty in exhaling, which indicates that the *kidney* is involved, for the *kidney* helps the *lung* respire, and protracted difficult respiration with prolonged exhalation is a sign of *kidney* impairment.

In summary, chronic bronchitis, within the system of Chinese medicine, is a disease impairing the *lung*, *spleen* and *kidney*. Exogenous pathogens play an important role only during acute exacerbations.

Accurate interpretation of the above traditional medical terms using modern medical concepts is very difficult, but a tentative comparison based on modern research of related traditional medical theories shows the similarities. The *kidney* is considered the foundation of the inborn constitution; impaired *kidney* is closely associated with genetic anomaly. The function of the *spleen* is closely related with immunity, including vulnerability to exogenous pathogens and allergic reactions. There are disparities, however, between the two systems of medicine so far as treatment is concerned.

In traditional Chinese medicine, treatment of chronic bronchitis is aimed chiefly at the *lung*, *spleen* and *kidney*. Various tonics in combination plus expectorants have been used clinically. Antitussives are only used when coughing is distressing, otherwise they are not recommended, because coughing up the phlegm helps to clear the airway obstruction. The unique theory and practice of traditional Chinese medicine in the treatment of chronic bronchitis has aroused the interest of many medical professionals, including Western-trained doctors in China. Controlled clinical trials using tonics (*lung*, *spleen* and *kidney* tonics) plus expectorants have shown promise in reducing or eliminating recurrence of the disease. The formula of *Guben Wan* (Pill for Strengthening the Constitution) tested by China Academy of Traditional Chinese Medicine can be taken as an example.

In long-term treatment (three to five years) of 140 cases of chronic bronchitis, 23 (16.4%) were clinically cured with no recurrence, 76 (54.3%) showed marked improvement and 26 (18.6%) improved; whereas in a control group in which the patients received only symptomatic treatment during acute exacerbations, none were clinically cured, 4.2% showed marked improvement and 33.3% improved.

The ingredients of the formula and their pharmacological actions are shown in Table IV-4. From this, it can be seen that the formula consists of tonics for the *lung*, *spleen* and *kidney* and some expectorants.

Table IV-4

Ingredients of *Guben Wan* **(Pill for Strengthening the Constitution) and Their Pharmacological Actions**

Ingredients	Actions
Radix Astragali (astragalus root)	A *lung* and *spleen* tonic for replenishing *qi*
Rhizoma Atractylodis Macrocephalae (white atractylodes rhizome)	Invigorates the function of the *spleen*
Radix Ledebouriellae (ledebouriella root)	A wind-dispelling drug for treating colds; combined with the above two ingredients forming "Jade Screen Powder" (cf. p.30)
Radix Codonopsis Pilosulae (pilose asiabell root)	Invigorates the function of the *spleen* to replenish *qi*
Poria	Invigorates the function of the *spleen* and removes dampness
Radix Glycyrrhizae (licorice)	Invigorates the function of the *spleen*'
Pericarpium Citri Reticulatae (tangerine peel)	An expectorant
Rhizoma Pinelliae (pinellia tuber)	An expectorant, particularly for cough with profuse thin phlegm
Fructus Psoraleae (psoralea fruit)	Invigorates the function of the *kidney*
Placenta Hominis (humen placenta)	Tonifies the *lung* and *kidney* for replenishing *qi*, blood and vital essence

Chronic Gastritis

Chronic gastritis is chronic inflammation of the gastric mucosa. This common disease affecting the digestive system accounts for 80-90%

of the cases that undergo gastroscopy in China. The diagnosis is predominantly based upon histological findings, which classify it into superficial and atrophic gastritis. In superficial gastritis, inflammatory cell infiltration is limited to the superficial half of the gastric mucosa, while the glands are preserved. Superficial gastritis may represent the initial stage in the development of the disease. In atrophic gastritis, which represents the next stage, inflammatory infiltration extends to the deep portions of the mucosa, and there is progressive distortion and destruction of the glands. As chronic gastritis progresses, there may be morphological changes of gastric glandular elements. The conversion of gastric glands to small-intestinal mucosal glands is called intestinal metaplasia.

Another classification (according to R. G. Strickland) is to divide chronic gastritis into two major forms (types A and B) based on the distribution of chronic inflammation in the gastric mucosa and other pathogentic implications. Type A gastritis is less common of the two. It characteristically involves the body and fundus of the stomach with relative sparing of the antrum and may occasionally lead to pernicious anemia. The frequent presence of antibodies to parietal cells of the stomach in sera of patients with type A gastritis has suggested an autoimmune pathogenesis for this form of gastritis. Type B gastritis is much more common; in younger patients it principally involves the antrum, whereas in older patients the entire stomach may be affected. Type B gastritis has been shown to have a strong association with Helicobacter pylori infection. Chronic reflux of bile has also been proposed as a potential factor in the genesis of type B.

Since the risk of stomach cancer in patients with chronic gastritis is much higher than that of the general population, many Chinese researchers have engaged in traditional treatment of this disease.

The most common symptom of chronic superficial gastritis is epigastric pain accompanied by distention, which is aggravated by eating cold or indigestible food. Anorexia, lassitude, and belching are also common. According to the principles of traditional Chinese medicine, in most cases the diagnosis is weakness (*qi* deficiency) of the *spleen* and stomach associated with cold syndrome or perverse flow of *qi*.

Patients with chronic atrophic gastritis usually have similar complaints. Atrophic lesions of the gastric mucosa can be considered blood stasis from the traditional medical point of view. A high incidence of clinical manifestations, such as purple or dark gums and lower lip, has been reported in most chronic atrophic cases.

Traditional treatment is therefore aimed at reinforcing the function of the *spleen* and stomach with appropriate tonics. Ingredients for warming the stomach and restoring the normal flow of *qi* (such as relieving belching) are often added for superficial gastritis, while ingredients for removing blood stasis are added for atrophic gastritis.

Jishuitan Hospital in Beijing used a herbal formula of granules called *Weining* on 408 patients with chronic superficial gastritis diagnosed by fibrogastroscopy and histology. The patients were divided into two groups: 325 patients received 20g of *Weining* three times a day for three months, and 83 patients received a placebo. The study was carried out as a single blind trial. In the first group, the symptomatic, gastroscopic and histologic effective rates were 90.5%, 81.9% and 72.8% respectively, while in the placebo group they were 50.6%, 46.3% and 16.7% respectively.

Weining consists of the following ingredients:

Radix Codonopsis Pilosulae (pilose asiabell root)— a *qi* tonic which invigorates the function of *spleen* and stomach.

Poria— a stomachic.

Rhizoma Atractylodis Macrocephalae (white atractylodes rhizome)— a *qi* tonic which invigorates the function of the *spleen* and stomach.

Radix Aucklandiae (aucklandia root)— a carminative for relieving epigastric distention and belching.

Fructus Meliae Toosendan (Sichuan Chinaberry)— a carminative for relieving epigastric pain.

Fructus Mume (black plum)— an astringent.

Experiments have shown that *Weining* protects the gastric mucous membrane in rats and guinea pigs. Its effect is similar to that of Cimetidin in drug-induced gastritis. It also inhibits pepsin secretion.

As for chronic atrophic gastritis, there have been quite a few studies with promising results. Qindao Navy Sanatorium and another hospital looked at 910 cases of atrophic gastritis, in which most (863 cases) were type B atrophic gastritis. Four hundred and thirty-eight cases were accompanied by metaplasia of the intestinal mucosa. All the patients were treated with a herbal decoction, containing primarily Radix Astragali (a large dose of 30g daily), Cortex Cinnamomi 10g, Fructus Evodiae 10g, Fructus Aurantii 10g, Rhizoma Curcumae Longae 10g, Rhizoma Ligustici Chuanxiong 10g, Flos Carthami 10g, Semen

Persicae 10g, Radix Salviae Miltiorrhizae 30g, Rhizoma Sparganii 10g, Rhizoma Zedoariae 10g, and Radix Glycyrrhizae 6g. Radix Astragali and Radix Glycyrrhizae are *qi* tonics which invigorate the function of the *spleen* and stomach, Cortex Cinnamomi and Fructus Evodiae dispel cold and warm the stomach. The rest are used for eliminating blood stasis.

After treatment with the decoction, all 910 were re-examined by gastroscopy and biopsy. Six hundred and thirty-seven (70%) were basically cured: the symptoms were eliminated, atrophied glands restored and intestinal epithelial metaplasia reversed on biopsy, gastroscopy also showed normal appearance of gastric mucosa; 245 cases (26.9%) improved, and 28 cases (3.1%) showed no change. The side effects of the decoction are very mild in long-term administration. Only a few patients felt dizzy, and the reaction was easily alleviated by adding Cortex Moutan Radicis.

Diabetes Mellitus

Diabetes mellitus has afflicted human beings for thousands of years. More than 2,000 years ago, *Canon of Medicine* described a disease manifested by polyphagia and polydipsia named *xiaoke* (消渴),of which *xiao* (消) means "ever hungry," and *ke* (渴) means "ever thirsty." *Canon of Medicine* says: "This disease is often encountered in obese individuals who have taken too much fatty and sweet food." In the second century A.D., Zhang Zhongjing, the most famous physician of the time, described *xiaoke* as "a disease characterized by polyuria despite dire thirst" and recommended a kidney tonic formula called *Shen Qi Wan* (Pill for Replenishing Kidney *Qi*) as treatment. At present this formula is still used to treat diabetes mellitus. In the sixth century A.D., Zhen Liyan recorded the sweetness of *xiaoke* patients' urine in his book *Gu Jin Lu Yan Fang* (*Records of Ancient and Modern Recipes*). He described *xiaoke* as "a disease marked by thirst, polydipsia, polyuria and sweet urine." Sweet urine in *xiaoke* was thereafter repeatedly described in ancient medical literature.

From the above discussion, it can be concluded that *xiaoke* is roughly equivalent to diabetes mellitus, though it may have included other diseases such as diabetes insipitus. *Xiaoke* was diagnosed primarily on the basis of symptoms and seldom on the sweetness of urine due to the lack of laboratory tests at that time.

The etiology and pathogenesis of diabetes mellitus based on what we knew about *xiaoke* can be considered in the following ways:

The causes of diabetes mellitus are: constitutional defect (usually a defect manifested by *yin* deficiency), improper diet (eating too much, particularly sweet food and wine), and depressed emotions (particularly anger and melancholy). All may lead to a *yin* deficiency with dryness and heat.

Most of the symptoms in diabetes mellitus can be attributed to *yin* deficiency with accompanying dryness-heat or fire. Dire thirst with polydipsia and dryness of the mouth and throat are manifestations of *yin* deficiency of the *lung* and stomach with impairment of body fluids (dryness); increased appetite, polyphagia and emaciation, often accompanied by constipation, are manifestations of *yin* deficiency of the stomach with exuberant activity (fire) of the stomach manifested by increased appetite. Polyuria accompanied by sweet urine and weakness of the loins and knees is due to deficiency of *kidney yin*. The basic pathogenesis of diabetes mellitus is therefore deficiency of the *lung*, stomach and *kidney*. Dryness-heat or fire is secondary to *yin* deficiency, but different visceral organs (*lung*, stomach or *kidney*) may be predominately involved. Diabetics also often complain about loss of strength and lassitude, which indicates deficiency of *qi*.

Dietotherapy was first emphasized for treatment of *xiaoke*. Wang Tao pointed out in his book *Wai Tai Mi Yao* (*Medical Secrets of an Official*) (752 A.D.): "*Xiaoke* patients should abstain from flour, fat meat, rice and fruit." Physical activity was also recommended. Wang Tao advised: "Do not lie down immediately after a heavy meal, and do not sit all day long.... Appropriate physical activity is necessary, though patients should avoid overfatigue and must not be forced to do what is beyond their capacity." He also advised patients to walk after each meal. These principles still hold today.

So far as herbal treatment is concerned, a great variety of herbs and formulae have been recorded in the literature. Based on the above pathogenesis, the majority of herbs used are tonics, most of which replenish *yin* and/or *qi*, and some of which relieve dryness-heat and/or eliminate fire. Only two formulae and the individual herbs most commonly used and proven to have a hypoglycemic action are listed below:

Compound formulae:

Jiang Tang Jia Pian (Tablet for Reducing Blood Sugar No. A) is composed of Radix Astragali (astragalus root), Rhizoma Polygonati (Siberian solomonseal rhizome), Radix Psudostellariae (psudostellaria root), Radix Rehmanniae (rehmannia), and Radix Trichosanthis (trichosanthes root).

Xiao Ke Ping Pian (Tablet for Relieving *Xiaoke*) is composed of Radix Astragali (astragalus root), Radix Ginseng (ginseng), Radix Trichosanthis (trichosanthes root), Radix Asparagi (asparagus root), Rhizoma Anemarrhenae (anemarrhena rhizome), and Radix Puerariae (pueraria root).

Reports on these two formulae have shown an effective rate of 75-80% in the treatment of non-insulin-dependent diabetes mellitus. So far there are no definite findings on herbal treatment of insulin-dependent diabetes mellitus.

Individual herbs:

Yin tonics : Fructus Corni (dogwood fruit); Fructus Mori (mulberry).

Qi tonics: Radix Ginseng (ginseng), Radix Astragali (astragalus root).

Herbs to relieve heat and fire: Rhizoma Coptidis (coptis root), Radix Scutellariae (scutellaria root).

Others: Radix Puerariae (Pueraria root), Cortex Mori Radicis (mulberry bark), Momordica charantia.

The mechanisms of hypoglycemic action of the herbs may vary. For example, Radix Ginseng greatly reduces blood sugar in male rats with alloxan diabetes, but the effect is toned down in female rats. Rhizoma Coptidis has no effect on insulin secretion and release; its hypoglycemic effect may be glyconeogenesis and/or glycolysis. Momordica charantia seems to have similar antigenicity and bioactivity with insulin, for its extract can combine with insulin receptors and insulin antibodies.

Hyperthyroidism

Hyperthyroidism is a syndrome of sustained hyperfunction of the thyroid that can originate in a variety of ways. Common manifestations include nervousness, emotional agitation, inability to sleep, palpitations, loss of strength, tremors, frequent bowel movements, excessive sweating and intolerance to heat. Weight loss is usual despite a well-maintained or increased appetite. In most cases a goiter can be found.

In traditional Chinese medicine, though there was no such term as hyperthyroidism, goiters were well recorded. Hyperthyroidism was recently linked to goiter and treated with Sargassum (seaweed) and Thallus Laminariae seu Eckloniae (laminaria or ecklonia) as recommended in the ancient literature, but results were disappointing. Though usually effective at first, after a couple of weeks all the symptoms returned, including elevation of serum T3 and T4 levels despite continuation of the treatment. Analysis showed the high percentage of iodide in these drugs. It is known in Western medicine that iodide inhibits the release of hormones from the hyperfunctioning thyroid gland. Its ameliorative effects occur rapidly, but the response to iodide alone is often incomplete and transient.

In terms of traditional medical theory, the pathogenesis of hyperthyroidism can be analyzed as follows: Although hyperthyroidism is characterized by excess production of the thyroid hormone, it should not be taken as an excess syndrome in the traditional sense if all clinical manifestations are considered. Some of the symptoms such as irritability, palpitation, insomnia and intolerance to heat may be attributed to "endogenous fire" (cf. Chapter I), but they are the result of deficiency of *yin* which leads to relative exuberance of *yang* with "fire" manifestations. Other symptoms such as loss of strength and excessive sweating are manifestations of deficiency of *qi*. Hyperthyroidism should therefore be diagnosed primarily as a deficiency syndrome and treated with tonics. Treatment with Sargassum and Thallus Laminariae seu Eckloniae is aimed merely at reducing the goiter; it eliminates rather than tonifies.

Recently there have been a number of reports on tonic treatment of hyperthyroidism with satisfactory results. The report from Shanghai College of Traditional Chinese Medicine demonstrates the therapeutic effect of Radix Astragali in a randomized controlled study. The basic formula they used contains the following ingredients: Radix Astragali 30-45g, Radix Paeoniae Alba 12g, Radix Rehmanniae 15g, Rhizoma Cyperi 12g, Spica Prunellae 30g, and Radix Polygoni Multiflori 20g. Tonics are predominant: Radix Astragali is a *qi* tonic used in great quantity; Radix Paeoniae, Radix Rehmanniae and Radix Polygoni Multifori are *yin* tonics; Spica Prunellae is a herb for eliminating the goiter, and Rhizoma Cyperi is a carminative (a drug which normalizes the flow of *qi*) used to soothe the *liver* (irritability and emotional agitation are believed to be due to stagnation of *qi* in the *liver*).

Of the 98 patients treated with this decoction (for six months to three years), 61 (62.2%) were cured, showing normal radioiodine uptake and normal serum T_3 and T_4 levels; 19 (19.4%) showed marked improvement, and 8 (8.2%) some improvement. Forty-five patients were checked six months to four years after the treatment; 43 of those were symptom-free with normal serum T_3 and T_4 levels.

In order to study the effect of Radix Astragali, 56 patients with hyperthyroidism were randomly divided into two groups: One group received the above decoction, and the other received the above decoction without Radix Astragali. Symptoms were alleviated in both, but only those who received Radix Astragali had marked reduction in serum T_3 and T_4 levels.

Male Infertility

Male infertility is the cause of childlessness in a third of the couples who wish to have children. In Western medicine, the causes are multifarious, but in many cases the cause cannot be found, and infertility is diagnosed as idiopathic with defective spermatogenesis. There is a great deal of controversy over hormone treatment.

In traditional Chinese medicine, defective spermatogenesis is believed to be due to deficiency of the *kidney yin*, for the *kidney yin* chiefly refers to vital essence, including reproductive essence: in male it is semen. A great number of formulae have been recorded in traditional medical literature. One still widely used today is called *Wu Zi Yan Zong Wan*, which means "Pills of Five Kinds of Seeds (or Fruits) for Bringing Forth Offspring." It consists of the following ingredients: Semen Cuscutae (dodder seed), Fructus Schisandrae (schisandra fruit), Fructus Lycii (wolfberry fruit), Fructus Rubi (raspberry fruit) and Semen Plantaginis (plantain seed).

Shen from Nanjing College of Traditional Chinese Medicine reported on 100 cases of male infertility treated with the above formula combined with additional ingredients, such as Radix Rehmanniae, Radix Codonopsis Pilosulae, and Radix Angelicae Sinensis. Of the 100 patients, there were 46 with seminal abnormality, which included reduced density and low motility of sperm; 47 with aspermia; and 7 with seminal fluid totally devoid of sperm. After treatment, 82 were cured and the wives of 45 became pregnant.

In our institute, the effect of *Wu Zi Yan Zong Wan* was studied on rats. Old male rats of the same age (16 months) were randomly divided into two groups: One group was given extract of *Wu Zi Yan Zong Wan* by gavage daily for three weeks, and the control group was given the same quantity of tap water. Each was then mated with a young female rat four months old. Three-fourths of the female rats mated with the *Wu Zi Yan Zong Wan* group got pregnant, while only one-fourth of those mated with the control group got pregnant. The homogenate of each rat's epididymis was examined. Both the number and motility of sperms of *Wu Zi Yan Zong Wan* group were much greater than those of the control group.

CHAPTER V

TRADITIONAL CHINESE MEDICINE AND THE AGING

Gerontology is a special branch of traditional Chinese medicine. Priority was given to this branch of medicine not only for the sake of the common people, but because emperors of the past dynasties wished to live forever. They appointed physicians and alchemists to study the art and develop medicines for this purpose.

Paying respect to the aged is part of the traditional ethic of the Chinese people. Even emperors in the past conducted various activities to show their respect. For example, in 1785, Emperor Qianlong of the Qing Dynasty invited more than 3,000 old people to a banquet in the imperial court. The emperor himself proposed a toast to those over 90 years of age, and the oldest, at 105 years, was treated as an official of the highest rank. The emperor poured his wine for him. After the banquet the guests were given walking sticks, embroidered silk, fur coats, and antiques.

Chinese traditional gerontology has its own unique theories and experience. As a branch of medicine, it can be traced back to the 2,000-year-old *Canon of Medicine* (also called *Yellow Emperor's Internal Classic*), the oldest and greatest medical classic extant in China. There, pathogenesis of aging and the rules for preserving health are recorded. Using this as a basis, experiences have been accumulated, many of which are still popular today. According to the latest statistics, there are more than 5 million people over the age of 80 in mainland China, among whom the oldest is a woman 116 years of age. Longevity is certainly the result of many factors, maintaining health in the later years being one of the most important.

Basic Features of Aging

Canon of Medicine says that the natural life span is one hundred years. According to *Yang Sheng Lun* (*Treatise on Health Preservation*), a book written in the third century A.D., the maximum life span for human beings is 120 years. Modern estimates based on division of pulmonary fibroblasts put the span of human life at about 110 years.

Physiologic decline is the characteristic feature of aging. Even in healthy older adults whose physiologic functions are maintained, functional decrements occur in most organ systems. Expressed in traditional medical terms, most visceral functions are weakened; the *yin-yang* balance is thus maintained at a lower level, which means reduced homeostasis and capacity for adaptation to the external environment.

Among the visceral organs, the *kidney* is often considered most important as it is in charge of growth, development, reproduction and aging. Apart from urine secretion and micturition, the *kidney* is closely related with bone metabolism, brain activity, control of skillful actions, and sensitivity of the ear. Its function is reflected in the hair, for growth of hair depends upon the vital essence stored in the *kidney*. Therefore, loss of reproductive ability, memory impairment, whitening of the hair, loosening of the teeth, reduction of hearing, and bone changes in the aged are all attributed to diminished function of the *kidney*.

Cause of Senility

Aging cannot be prevented, and increasing feebleness of body and mind is inevitable. However, premature weakening and inability to live one's full life span are not natural. The causes of senility are of two types: innate and acquired.

Those born with a strong constitution may live a longer life than those without, but traditional Chinese medicine stresses that innate factors are not fixed since birth. They can be changed under the influence of acquired factors. According to traditional medical theory, inborn nature is handed down from generation to generation by the "vital essence." Before birth, "vital essence" refers to the parents' sperm and ovum. After birth, it is stored in the *kidney* and regulates growth, development and functioning of various visceral organs. Excessive consumption of vital essence will result in a deficit, similar to an inborn shortage, while proper protection and cultivation will compensate for an inborn shortage.

Approaches to Prevent Senility and Retard Aging

There are two main purposes in the practices of traditional Chinese health preservation: to prevent feebleness of the body and mind incidental to old age, and to retard the process of aging to prolong the life span. The main approaches are as follows:

I. Adaptation to Nature

The relevant adaptation of a human being to the natural environment is a basic theory in traditional Chinese medicine. According to this idea, the physical structure and physiological functioning of the human body must conform to the variations in the natural environment. One must adapt to climatic changes and circadian alternations.

An important aspect of adaptation to nature is alternation of being awake and sleep. One should keep a regular life, sleeping at night and working in the day. A nap at noon is necessary for those in their later years. This is called "night and noon sleep." It is said in Chinese gerontology that good sleep is better than a wonderful recipe for preserving health and prolonging life.

Warmth in spring, heat in summer, coolness in autumn and coldness in winter — all influence the functional processes of the human body. Another important way to adapt to nature is to match the method of health preservation to the season with, for example, the diet. According to *Yin Shan Zheng Yao* (*Principles of Correct Diet*) "Food made of flour is good for spring because it is cool in nature; food made of beans is good for summer because many of the beans are cold in nature; food made of sesame is good for autumn because it can relieve dryness; and food made of broomcorn millet is good for winter because it is hot in nature."

II. Maintenance of a Calm and Cheerful Mood

In traditional Chinese medicine, the relationship between emotion and the visceral organs is stressed. Normal emotions are beneficial to the physiological processes of visceral organs, while emotional agitation usually impairs their functioning, resulting in disease and premature senility.

In order to avoid emotional agitation, one must know how to exercise self-control and maintain a calm and cheerful mood. In that the Taoist concept of human conduct was frequently emphasized in the literature about Chinese gerontology, the aged are advised to let things take their own course so as to avoid trouble.

III. Rational Diet

A rational diet is the first guarantee for health and longevity. It is stressed in traditional Chinese medicine that food should be diversified; partiality to a special kind of food may be harmful to health. It is better to have diet of multiple ingredients including meat, cereals, vegetables and fruit. *Canon of Medicine* recommended a "balanced diet" to the aged more than 2,000 years ago. "Cereals are the principal food; various kinds of fruit, meat and vegetables should also be taken in proper proportion." "Cereals, meat, fruit and vegetables should be taken according to the requirements for proper nourishment; eating to excess is harmful."

As each flavor produces a different chemical reaction in the body, different tastes should be prepared in appropriate proportions. The principles of Chinese cookery create food not only delicious but also conducive to good health. The literature says: "Sour overcomes spicy hot — vinegar added to spicy food makes the hot taste mild and lessens the dryness; sweet moderates the sour — sugar added to sour food lessens the sour taste and its astringent action." Overall, food should not be too sour, too sweet, too pungent, nor too salty.

It is also stressed that food should be taken at regular intervals in appropriate amounts. Excessive hunger and overeating should be avoided and fat restricted. It is advised to chew the food well before swallowing. Warm soft food is usually preferred, and cold, hard and glutinous food that is apt to cause digestive disorders should be avoided. A vegetarian diet without much salt is advised.

The famous physician Sun Simiao (581-682), an expert in gerontology who lived over 100 years, advised the following: "Take a short walk after each meal. Lying down after eating will result in various diseases." "After each meal rub the face and knead the abdomen with the hands to promote secretion of digestive juice." This valuable advice has been adopted by many old people. A popular folk proverb says: Walking 100 paces after each meal, and you'll live to 99.

Alcoholic drinks and tea are related to diet. The Chinese were making wine four or five thousand years ago. As one of the oldest and most important medicines used in ancient times, the character for "medicine" (醫) contains the radical for "wine" (酉). Alcohol helps

85

promote blood circulation and dispel cold. It is often used in the processing of herbs to enhance their efficacy. A small amount of alcohol is beneficial to the health of the aged, for it "counteracts pathogens, increases blood flow, promotes digestion and dispels depression; but the quantity should be restricted" (*Principles of Correct Diet*).

Tea originated in China. It was recorded in writing as early as the seventh century B.C.; since the sixth century A.D., drinking tea has become a popular habit all over China. It is stated in *Shen Nong's Herbal* that tea is bitter in taste and cold in nature, and regular consumption will make one nimble and enjoy a good life.

There are three categories of tea according to the method of processing. Green tea is non-fermented, Wulong tea is half-fermented, and black tea is fully fermented. From the point of view of traditional Chinese medicine, green tea is cool in nature, and may be used for antiinflammatory and detoxifying purposes. Black tea is somewhat warm, and may promote digestion and arrest diarrhea. Wulong tea is between the two and most appropriate for daily use. Recent research has shown that tea acts to regulate lipid metabolism, reduce blood cholesterol, and alleviate accumulation of lipids in the vascular wall to maintain normal elasticity of blood vessels. It is therefore useful to treat obesity and prevent cardiovascular disease. The aged, however, are advised to dilute their tea, for strong tea increases the heart beat and urine excretion, and disturbs regular sleep if taken in the evening. Strong tea should be avoided by those with constipation, for its astringent action may aggravate the condition.

The proper way to make tea is worth mentioning. Water just begun to boil will produce a good flavorful infusion. If the water has been boiled too long, all the carbon dioxide will be evaporated, and the flavor, color and taste of the tea will be damaged.

Dietotherapy, another issue related to diet, is particularly emphasized in traditional Chinese medicine for treating chronic diseases in the aged. It is discussed in detail in Chapter IX.

IV. Preservation of Vital Essence

The so-called vital essence is considered the source of life and basic material for life activity. There are two kinds of vital essence in the human body: innate essence and acquired essence. Both are believed to be stored in the *kidney* and called "*kidney* essence." Acquired essence is chiefly derived from food, and innate essence is derived from the reproductive essence (the sperm and ovum) of the parents. As they are interdependent, the innate essence needs constant nourishment from the acquired essence. An embryo formed from the fusion of the parents' reproductive essence turns into the innate essence of the embryo and then the fetus. After birth, essence is then acquired from food. Both the inherited innate essence and that derived from food constitute the vital essence of the *kidney*, which makes possible growth and development.

When a certain age is reached, part of the *kidney* essence will turn into reproductive essence; according to *Canon of Medicine*, the female at 14 will begin menstruation, and the male at 16 will be able to have seminal discharge, both signifying the power of reproduction. The unique view in traditional Chinese medicine is that the reproductive essence not only gives rise to the formation of innate essence in the offspring, but also influences one's own innate essence. The innate essence is therefore constantly changing through nourishment by acquired essence from food and replenishment by the production of reproductive essence.

Preservation of vital essence refers to the prevention of excessive discharge of reproductive essence. Traditional Chinese medical principles emphasize that sexual overindulgence is not only harmful to health but will make longevity impossible. This is particularly important for the aged. Sun Simiao gave the following advice: "Those who wish to preserve their life must first preserve their vital essence." "Those over forty who refrain from discharging vital essence usually live long lives." "A man over sixty should abstain from seminal discharge unless he has a strong physique." Sexual moderation does not mean asceticism. Regarding the proper frequency of intercourse, Sun suggested: "For those in their twenties, once every four days, for those in their fifties, once every twenty days, for those in their sixties, no seminal discharge is advised or once every month if they are still strong enough."

V. Health-preserving Exercises

Traditional exercises for preserving health are different from modern physical exercises. They include *qigong*, *taijiquan* (a kind of traditional Chinese shadow boxing), massage, teeth tapping and others.

Both inner cultivating *qigong* and roborant *qigong* are commonly practiced by the aged (cf. Chapter VIII). It has been revealed that those who practice *qigong* have better vision and hearing, and fairer hair and skin than others of the same age. Physical movement, memory, appetite and sleeping patterns are also superior in the former group. An altered estradiol/testosterone ratio in the aged tends to turn to normal after one year's practice of *qigong*. The activity of superoxide dismutase is also markedly increased after *qigong* practice.

The name *taiji* originates from the Chinese classic *Yi Jing* (*Book of Changes*). *Taiji* means the origin or basic element of all kinds of matter. *Taijiquan* is a kind of Chinese boxing characterized by gentle, slow and continuous movements, in which the mind is highly concentrated and breathing deep, prolonged, even and quiet. In that it promotes activity of the central nervous system and improves the function of visceral organs, it is particularly appropriate for the aged to build up their health.

Teeth tapping, known as the "secret to longevity," was one of the health preservation exercises introduced by Sun Simiao. The procedure is quite simple. In the morning and evening tap the upper and lower teeth together. The molars, incisors and canines should be tapped separately because they are not on the same horizontal plane. After tapping, lick the gums and buccal mucosa with the tip of the tongue to stimulate secretion of saliva. Gargle with the saliva and swallow it. Then, massage the gums with the tongue, grit the teeth and puff out the cheeks to increase salivary secretion. Swallow the saliva in several gulps. This procedure is helpful for strengthening the teeth which are necessary for sound digestion.

VI. Herbal Medication

Traditional Chinese medicine has a long history dealing in herbal medication for preserving health, preventing senility and promoting longevity. In *Shen Nong's Herbal*, among the 365 species of herbs listed, 165 were recorded to deal with the above. In later centuries, more "anti-aging" herbs and formulae were studied and recorded. The imperial court of the Qing Dynasty (1644-1911) paid particular attention to investigations on retardation of aging and prevention of senility. Quite a few of these formulae have been handed down and are used today.

Recent research on ancient "anti-aging" herbs and formulae has shown the effect of these drugs from the modern perspective:

Radix Ginseng (ginseng, root of Panax ginseng C. A. Mey) enhances the capacity of physical and mental activities, and particularly improves concentration, thinking and memory. It has an "adaptogen" effect, increasing the adaptability of the body to guard against various harmful stimuli, physical, chemical or biological. In animal experiments, it has been shown to stimulate the pituitary-adrenocortical system and sexual glands, both in the male and female. It prevents hypercholesterolemia and atherosclerosis. It contains prostisol, which promotes biosynthesis of protein, DNA and RNA. Saponin derived from Panax ginseng fruit has been shown to improve memory and senility, increase plasma testosterone and lower estradiol in older males; it also reduces physiological age based on various functional indices.

Radix Astragali (astragalus, root of Astragalus membranaceus Bge.) enhances the immune function, including phagocytosis of reticuloendothelial cells and production of immunoglobulins. It also increases the production of interferon induced by virus. As it is actually an immuno-modulator, it suppresses the immune function in cases of hyperimmunity. It promotes protein metabolism and has a remarkable effect on the growth of diploid cells in the human embryo lung, retarding natural aging and increasing the life span of cells to 98 generations (compared to 61-66 generations in the control group).

Rhizoma Polygonati (Siberian solomonseal rhizome) has been shown to prolong the average life span of silkworms by about 39%.

Though not a herb, margarite (pearl) is frequently used in Chinese herbal medication. It has been shown to prolong the life span of silkworms, inhibit accumulation of lipofuscin in mice, and improve the memory of older people.

More research has been done on the compound formulae recorded in ancient medical literature and later modifications. The following is a partial list: *Gui Ling Ji* (Elixir of Life), made of Cornu Cervi Pantotrichum (pilose deerhorn), Hippocampus (sea·horse), Herba Epimedii (epimedium) and Radix Ginseng (ginseng) as the chief ingredients; *Qing Gong Shou Tao Wan* (Qing Court Longevity Pill) which contains Radix Rehmanniae (rehmannia root), Fructus Lycii (wolfberry fruit), Fructus Alpiniae Oxyphyllae (bitter cardamon) and Semen Juglandis (walnut); *Huan Jing Jian* (Essence-restoring Decoction), made of Radix Rehmanniae, Semen Astragali Complanati (flattened milkvetch seed), Herba Cynomorii (cynomorium), Semen Cuscutae (dodder seed) and Radix Polygoni Multiflori (fleeceflower root); *Qing Gong Chang Chun Dan* (Qing Court Ever-youth Pill), made of Cortex Eucommiae (eucommia bark), Radix Polygalae (polygala root), Rhizoma Acori

Graminei (grass-leaved sweetflag rhizome) and Fructus Corni (dogwood fruit); and *Sheng Mai Ye* (Pulse-activating Solution), made of Radix Ginseng (ginseng), Radix Ophiopogonis (ophiopogon root) and Fructus Schisandrae (schisandra fruit).

Most of these ingredients are tonics, particularly *kidney* tonics. Radix Rehmanniae, Fructus Lycii, Radix Polygoni Multiflori, Fructus Corni and Semen Astragali Complanati are all tonics to replenish *kidney yin* (vital essence); and Herba Epimedii, Cornu Cervi Paentotrichum and Semen Cuscutae are tonics to invigorate *kidney yang* (vital function).

The above formulae have been studied to determine the following: clinical alleviation of senile symptoms, improvement of intelligence, reduction of serum lipid peroxide and improvement of blood testosterone and estradiol levels in the aged.

The Institute for Integration of Traditional and Modern Medicines, Beijing Medical University, studied the effect of *Wu Zi Yan Zong Ye* (WZYZY, Solution of Five Kinds of Seeds for Bringing Forth Offspring), an extract of *Wu Zi Yan Zong Wan* (Pills of Five Kinds of Seeds for Bringing Forth Offspring), one of the best known *kidney* tonic formulae for replenishing vital essence (cf. Chapter IV). Eighty men, aged 60-80, suffering from symptoms of senility but no other definable disease, were selected from a group of 472 old people in a community. The symptoms were: general weakness, intolerance to cold, aching in the loins and heels, loss of memory, tinnitus and incontinence of urine.

Table V-1

Plasma LPO, Erythrocyte SOD, Plasma T and E_2 Levels in Healthy Young Men and Old Men Without Disease Except Senility

Group	Number of individuals	LPO (nmol/ml)	SOD (μg/g Hb)	T (ng/dl)	E_2 (pg/ml)	E_2/T
Young	33	2.95±0.64	681.6±63.5	612.4±133.7	33.0±9.1	0.057±0.021
Old	80	4.48±0.72*	489.6±50.2*	476.2±140.8*	34.0±11.7	0.075±0.029*

* In comparison with the young individuals, $P < 0.01$.

Table V-2

Changes of Plasma LPO, Erythrocyte SOD, Plasma T and E₂ Levels in Old Men with Senility After Five-week Administration of WZYZY or Placebo*

Group		LPO (nmol/ml)	SOD (μg/g Hb)	T (ng/dl)	E₂ (pg/ml)	E₂/T
WZYZY	before treatment	4.49 +0.07	488.5 +46.5	473.8 +126.4	34.8 +10.1	0.071 +0.020
	after treatment	3.27 +0.52	571.4 +95.5	566.4 +116.8	32.6 +9.1	0.059 +0.018
Placebo	before treatment	4.48 +0.72	489.9 +57.4	480.3 +165.3	32.1 +8.9	0.073 +0.036
	after treatment	4.23 +0.62	503.4 +43.8	491.5 +132.6	34.4 +11.0	0.064 +0.024

They were divided into two random groups; one group was treated with WZYZY and the other was given a placebo. Five weeks later, there was marked clinical improvement in the WZYZY group but no change in the placebo group.

The plasma lipid peroxide (LPO), erythrocyte superoxide dismutase (SOD), plasma testosterone (T) and estradiol (E₂) levels were determined before treatment. In comparison with the 33 men in their twenties, LPO in the aged was much higher, SOD and T remarkably lower and the E₂/T ratio elevated.

By the end of the course of treatment, the plasma LPO was greatly reduced, SOD and T increased and E₂/T lowered in the WZYZY group, but there was no such change in the placebo group.

Animal experiments have also shown the effect of WZYZY. About 100 rats of various ages (2, 5, 10, 18 and 24 months; about 20 rats of each age) were divided into two groups at random, one group fed with WZYZY daily for five weeks, and the other group with a saline solution. Radioimmunoassay showed marked reduction of plasma T and elevation of E_2/T in the groups of 18 and 24 months fed with saline; in the corresponding age groups fed with WZYZY those levels were much better. There was no such obvious difference with the younger rats. This indicates that the herbal medicine used is different from testosterone preparations; it stimulates the sexual gland only when its function is diminished. The case with LPO seems to be different. Plasma LPO level was lower and erythrocyte SOD level higher in both younger and older rats fed with WZYZY than those of corresponding ages fed with the saline solution.

Though the research has shown how herbal formulae can improve the health of old adults, particularly those with symptoms of senility, there is still no direct evidence to prove their effect towards prolonging life. In most cases, non-medicinal measures are preferable to long-term medication.

CHAPTER VI
TRADITIONAL CHINESE MEDICINE IN THE TREATMENT OF CANCER

One of the great challenges facing traditional Chinese medicine is the treatment of cancer. Cancer is second to cardio- and cerebrovascular diseases as a cause of death in China and many other countries; it is natural to ask whether it can be treated by traditional medicine. This question is difficult to answer, because prognosis and treatment differ with each kind of cancer, its particular stage and the patient's constitution.

The history of cancer is probably as long as the history of mankind. The Chinese character for tumor appeared first in oracle-bone inscriptions of the 14th-11th century B.C. In medical literature, cancer was first described in *Zhou Hou Fang* (*A Handbook of Prescriptions for Emergencies*) compiled by Ge Hong (281-341 A.D.). He described cancer in the abdomen as "a mass which can be felt in the abdomen as hard as stone which causes such a severe stabbing pain, the patient cries day and night. Its gradual onset makes it difficult to uncover in the early stages. As it increases in size, emaciation follows. Prognosis is poor, and the patient usually dies within one hundred days."

Traditional Concept of Cancer

In the Chinese language, cancer is called *ai* (癌, derived from the character 嵒 which means rock). The first cancer so named was breast cancer, described in *Fu Ren Liang Fang* (*Effective Prescriptions for Women*), the comprehensive work on gynecology compiled by Chen Ziming in 1237. Chen wrote: "Due to depression or anger, a lump forms in the breast, which causes no pain or other symptoms at first. Many years later it becomes hard, the skin ulcerates and nipple retracts, like a rock with caverns. It is thus named *ai* of the breast."

The terms used in both Western and Chinese medicine for denoting malignant tumor indicate its morphological characteristics. The Chinese name is derived from the word for rock, describing the tumor's uneven surface and hard quality; cancer in English is derived from the Latin word for crab, symbolizing both the hardness and the dissemination of the tumor like a crab extending its legs outward. As regards etiology and pathogenesis of cancers in traditional Chinese medicine, although there have been many expositions for different kinds of cancer, it is not taken as a local disease; it is understood as a general disease with the tumor mass as a local manifestation. Common etiology includes "internal" and "external" causes. Internal causes are mostly constitutional and emotional. Cancer occurs frequently in the aged with weakened constitution and lowered body resistance, particularly in those with normal functioning of the body impaired by long-term emotional depression. External causes refer to various harmful factors in the external environment, such as toxic substances in food. Chronic stimulation is also stressed, for example, "excessive fried or roasted food eaten in a hurried way may cause lip cancer." Internal causes, particularly insufficient body resistance, is usually regarded as the primary cause.

All external causes can be taken as carcinogenic factors. Working over a long period of time when resistance is low will impair body function and bring about pathological changes. The most common change is local accumulation of stagnated blood, phlegm, damp, or toxic heat, which will give rise to the growth of cancer.

Pathological changes are recognized on the basis of clinical manifestations. Accumulation of phlegm is usually associated with the formation of hard nodular masses, particularly under the skin, such as enlarged lymph nodes in lymphoma or cancer metastasis. Damp is related to fluid discharge; in nasopharyngeal carcinoma, an accumulation of damp may be the cause of turbid nasal discharge. Toxic heat is usually encountered in the advanced stages or in cancer with secondary infection, manifested by fever, constipation and yellow tongue coating. Accumulation of stagnated blood or blood stasis is a common pathogenetic factor of tumors in the abdomen. This includes gynecological tumors, particularly if the mass is painful, palpable and tender. Another clinical feature of blood stasis is a purple tongue or purple dots or spots on the tongue. Since this phenomenon occurs so often, blood stasis is now considered a general pathogenetic mechanism for the growth of many kinds of cancer.

Among all the pathogenetic factors, lowered body resistance comes first. Classification of various deficiencies in body resistance has been discussed in Chapter II.

Compared with Western medicine, the above brief description of etiology and pathogenesis seems quite vague: It does not tell what specific function is impaired and what the stagnated blood, phlegm and toxic heat are. Traditional considerations, however, are still worth mentioning as they are closely related to treatment.

Herbal Medication of Cancer

The herbal drugs and formulae used in the treatment of cancer can be grouped into several modalities: therapies to strengthen body resistance, to clear toxic heat, to remove stagnated blood, to resolve phlegm, etc.

The crucial question is: Is traditional treatment really effective? The therapeutic efficacy of various herbs and formulae have been recorded and case studies done. However, due to historical restraints in cancer diagnosis and assessment of therapeutic effect, these records can only be taken as a clue to the modern use of traditional therapy; and due to possible spontaneous regression, though rare, reports of successful treatment in individual cases are insufficient to prove their effectiveness. It is therefore necessary to re-evaluate efficacy from a modern perspective with histological evidence and statistical analysis. In recent years, extensive studies have been carried out and encouraging results obtained with the following: (1) use of herbal medication as the sole form of treatment; (2) use of traditional therapy as an adjunct to surgical resection; (3) use of traditional therapy in combination with radiotherapy or chemotherapy.

I. Use of Herbal Medication as the Sole Form of Treatment

In this group of studies, most patients observed were those with nonresectable cancers. A comparative study was made in Longhua Hospital, Shanghai on herbal medication and chemotherapy of lung cancer. Sixty cases of advanced lung cancer (all of them squamous carcinoma as confirmed histologically) were divided into two groups: 30 cases were treated with herbal medication and 30 cases with chemotherapy. In the herbal medication group, the median survival period was 465 days

(12-month and 24-month survival rates were 66.7% and 13.3% respectively), while in the chemotherapy group, the median survival period was 204 days (12-month and 24-month survival rates were 33.3% and 3.3% respectively).

Similar results have been reported with primary liver cancer in the advanced stages. In a series of 112 cases, the half-year and one-year survival rates were 43.3% and 20% respectively in the herbal medication group; 20.8% and 8.3% respectively in the radiotherapy group; and 20% and 0% in the chemotherapy group. In the latter two groups, all the patients were of stage II, while in the herbal medication group, some patients were already in stage III.

It is probably more interesting to discuss the experimental studies of herbs used in the treatment of cancers. Among the therapies mentioned above, the following three have been widely studied:

1. Body-resistance-strengthening Therapy

In traditional treatment of cancer, therapies to strengthen body resistance are most strongly emphasized. Research has revealed that most drugs used to strengthen body resistance have some immunoenhancing action in cancer patients, particularly on cellular immunity (as demonstrated by increase of phagocytosis and T lymphocyte transformation rate). This therapy, so far as its therapeutic mechanism is concerned, can be thus taken as a kind of immunotherapy. (The action of body-resistance-strengthening therapy, as discussed in Chapter II, is far beyond immune enhancement or modulation.)

Practitioners of Western medicine have become increasingly interested in the use of immunotherapy for the treatment of cancer. It is based on the following premises: There is a host defense mechanism against cancer which is largely immunological in nature. Depression of this mechanism allows growth and spread of the cancer. Arrest of this immunosuppression will impair growth of the cancer. Though the theory sounds rational, there is some difficulty with clinical application due to lack of appropriate agents. The most widely used non-specific immunopotentiator agents in Western medicine are BCG, Corynebacterium parovum, and levamisole. Levamisole is an anthelmintic drug which can increase host resistance to tumor cells in some animal diseases, but its effect on cancer in humans has been disappointing. BCG and Corynebacterium increase the rate of survival in cancer patients, but both have side effects such as fever and hepatitis, which greatly limit their use. On the contrary, many herbs used to treat cancer have an immunoenhancing effect and no toxic or side effects.

2. Blood-stasis-removing Therapy

From the traditional medical point of view, treatment of cancer can be classified as either reinforcement of body resistance or elimination of pathogenic factors. Blood-stasis-removing therapy is of the latter category, for stagnated blood is seen as an important pathogenic factor in the growth of cancer. In Western medicine, cancer treatment is also classified in one of two categories: aggressive and supportive. Such classification does not suit traditional therapies, for the effect of body-resistance-strengthening is beyond merely supportive, and blood-stasis-removing may not be aggressive in nature.

Studies of cancer patients show that most suffer from hypercoagulability with microcirculatory disorders around the tumor. Drugs to remove blood stasis reduce blood coagulability and improve microcirculation, enabling immunocompetent cells to get into the tumor. Thus, elimination of cancer cells in blood-stasis-removing therapy is not directly due to the drug's aggression, so there are no such severe side effects as with aggressive treatment.

In the traditional treatment of cancer, blood-stasis-removing drugs were seldom used alone; they were almost always prescribed with herbs of other categories, such as body-resistance-strengthening herbs and toxic-heat-removing herbs. The results of experimental studies in this regard merit attention. Radix Salviae Miltiorrhizae (red sage root) is commonly used for removing blood stasis. An injection of red sage root extract in rats exaggerates the spontaneous pulmonary metastasis of cancer. However, when the root was combined with Rhizoma Atractylodis Macrocephalae (white atractylodes rhizome), a herbal drug to strengthen body resistance, there was no such exaggeration of cancer metastasis, and the animals survived longer than those which received no herbal treatment. It is thus advised to use blood-stasis-removing herbs in combination rather than as the sole form of treatment.

Besides improving local blood circulation, some blood-stasis-removing herbs work in other ways. For example, Radix Paeoniae Rubra (red peony root) is a commonly used herb for removing blood stasis. Both its water extract and ethyl alcoholic extract promote cancer metastasis in rats, but its butyl alcohol extract has a marked cancer-inhibiting effect. One herb may thus take on many actions.

3. Toxic-heat-clearing Therapy

Toxic heat in traditional Chinese medicine refers to pathogenic agents, usually infectious, which cause inflammation; drugs for eliminating toxic heat are thus usually used to treat infections and inflammations. Most have antipyretic, antibacterial or antiviral actions, while some enhance the immune function. This group of drugs is often used in the treatment of cancer, for cancer may manifest inflammation, especially when accompanied by secondary infection.

Dozens of herbs in this group have been found to have an anti-cancer effect in experiments and clinical trials either alone or in combination with chemotherapy. Their therapeutic mechanisms, though not yet clear, are multifarious. Some toxic-heat-eliminating herbs such as Radix Sophorae Subprostratae (subprostrate sophora root) impair nucleic acid metabolism of cancer cells. Others, such as Herba Oldenlandiae (oldenlandia), not only inhibit the growth of cancer cells, but also promote adreno-cortical activity and have a good effect when used in combination with chemotherapy. Others enhance the immune function of the host, or increase the antigenicity of the cancer cells, or improve local blood circulation.

Studies of toxic-heat-eliminating herbs have discovered some of their active components. Indirubin, used in the treatment of chronic leukemia, may serve as an example.

The Institute of Hematology, China Academy of Medical Sciences, used *Dang Gui Long Hui Wan* (Pill of Chinese Angelica, Gentian and Aloe) to treat chronic leukemia. The principal ingredients are Radix Angelicae Sinensis (Chinese angelica root), Radix Gentianae (Chinese gentian) and Aloe (aloes). Though the pill's effect on chronic granulocytic leukemia has been confirmed clinically, the results of pharmacologic study of the principal ingredients were discouraging: none of the three (Chinese angelica root, gentian or aloe) showed any anti-leukemic effect. Further analysis revealed that the active component was Indigo Naturalis (natural indigo), an auxiliary ingredient of the pill originally considered to be immaterial. Not only has the therapeutic effect of indigo to induce remission of chronic granulocytic leukemia been repeatedly confirmed, but its active agent — indirubin has been isolated and artificially synthesized. A study of 314 cases of chronic granulocytic leukemia treated with indirubin showed a total effective rate of 87.3%, with remission in 187 (59.5%) and improvement in 87 (27.7%). No side effect was found in about 60% of the cases; mild and moderate abdominal pain and diarrhea occurred in about 40%; suppression of bone marrow occurred in less than 5%. In comparison with busulphan (myleran), the most popular Western drug, indirubin apparently has less side effects or complications. The danger of bone marrow suppression is much greater with busulphan treatment.

II. Use of Traditional Therapy as an Adjunct to Surgical Resection

Surgical intervention is certainly the most effective treatment of cancer if resection is indicated, but only a small percentage of cancer patients can benefit from surgery. In many cases, spread of the tumor with metastasis renders radical resection impossible. Even when the tumor has been totally removed at the early stage, there is still danger of recurrence. This makes sense from the traditional medical point of view, which holds that cancer is not only a local lesion and that lowered body resistance is the primary cause. Removal of the tumor does not therefore ensure the patient is cured. Many whose tumors are removed at the early stage do enjoy a good prognosis. Removal of that burden influences the host-tumor relationship and allows recovery of resistance. However, restoration of body resistance depends largely upon the patient's constitution. Measures to improve the patient's constitution and body resistance are therefore an important part of the therapy.

In China, using herbal drugs to strengthen body resistance is widely practiced by medical professionals or patients themselves after surgical resection. With such therapy, not only does the patient recover quickly from surgery, but also the immune function, particularly cellular immunity, returns to normal. So far as immunological surveillance of cancer is concerned, reinforcing herbal therapy to enhance the cellular immunity is certainly advantageous.

Chemotherapy and/or radiotherapy is often used after removal of the tumor. In such cases, supplemental herbal medication also shows good results.

III. Use of Herbal Medication with Chemotherapy and/or Radiotherapy

Most of the drugs used in chemotherapy are cytotoxic. They are effective under certain conditions, such that their antitumor activity depends on the same properties that render them harmful to normal cells. Reduction of toxicity to normal cells and alleviation of adverse effects will make chemotherapy a more satisfactory treatment. The same is true of radiotherapy. In recent years, research has shown that herbal medication can reduce toxic and side effects of chemotherapy and radiotherapy, as well as enhance sensitivity to these therapies.

1. Reduction of Toxic and Side Effects of Chemotherapy and Radiotherapy

Evaluation of herbal medication in the treatment of cancer usually requires long-term observation, but assessment of toxic and side effect reduction with chemotherapy and radiotherapy is not so complicated. Herbal medication with chemotherapy or radiotherapy has thus become part of the routine regimen in many hospitals in China. In some hospitals, herbal medication is resorted to when toxic and side effects of the chemotherapy and radiotherapy appear.

The common toxic and side effects of chemotherapy are as follows:

(1) General weakness with lassitude, cardiac palpitation and shortness of breath;

(2) Digestive disturbances such as loss of appetite, nausea, vomiting or diarrhea;

(3) Bone marrow suppression, which is usually manifested as reduction of white blood cells and blood platelets.

There are many formulae of herbal medicine that can be used to correct the above disorders, and each clinician has her or his own preference. The formula used in China Academy of Traditional Chinese Medicine, which has been studied in many hospitals and widely recognized, is taken as one example.

This institution and more than 20 hospitals around China looked at the results of a granule preparation made from Radix Codonopsis Pilosulae (pilose asiabell root) 10g, Rhizoma Atractylodis Macrocephalae (white atractylodes rhizome) 10g, Fructus Lycii (wolfberry fruit) 15g, Semen Cuscutae (dodder seed) 15g, Fructus Ligustri Lucidi (lucid ligustrum fruit) 15g, and Fructus Psoraleae (psoralea fruit) 10g. Nine hundred and ninety-six patients with advanced stomach cancer were observed from 1983 to 1990. They were divided into two groups (test group and control group) on admission into the hospital for chemotherapy. In all cases, mitomycin, five-fluorouracil and vincristine were administered by intravenous drip. The above granule preparation was given orally to the test group twice a day in addition to chemotherapy; in the control group, patients received only chemotherapy. The six-week course of chemotherapy was completed in 94.44% of the test group, but in only 73.73% of the control group. Impairment of general condition, digestive disturbances and deterioration of blood were much milder in the test group. The assay of immune function also gave better results in the test group.

The toxic and side effects of radiotherapy are approximately the same as those of chemotherapy, but the former often includes symptoms of toxic heat such as fever. Thus in herbal treatment, ingredients to eliminate toxic heat are usually added.

Another point worth mentioning is the prevention and treatment of fibrosis induced by radiotherapy. Pneumonitis with consequent fibrosis is a common complication of radiation in the treatment of breast cancer and various intrathoracic organs. Radiation fibrosis may lead to a permanent loss of lung volume. Fibrosis and scar formation is taken as a manifestation of blood stasis in traditional Chinese medicine. One of the pharmacological actions of blood-stasis-removing herbs is to inhibit the formation of fibrous tissue. This has not only been demonstrated in animal experiments, but has been shown by successful clinical treatment of keloids after burn and corneal opacity from scar formation. The preventive and therapeutic effects of radiation fibrosis have also been shown in animal experiments.

Apart from herbal medication, acupuncture and moxibustion are used to treat toxic and side effects of chemotherapy and radiotherapy. They not only relieve symptoms such as nausea and vomiting, and improve the appetite, but also counteract bone marrow suppression. There was a recent study on acupuncture and moxibustion treatment of leukopenia induced by chemotherapy. In Henan Tumor Hospital and Henan College of Traditional Chinese Medicine, treatment of chemotherapy-induced leukopenia (with white blood cell count less than $4.0 \times 10^9/L$ or $4,000/mm$) was observed in 376 patients with malignant tumor. They were divided into three groups: the first group was treated with warming needling (a procedure that combines needling and moxibustion by attaching an ignited moxa stub to an inserted needle); the second group was treated with moxa cone moxibustion; and the third group was treated with an oral administration of the Western drugs batiol and leucogen to promote regeneration of white blood cells. After nine days, the white cell count had increased over $4 \times 10^9/L$ in 88.4% of the warming needling group, in 90.9% of the moxibustion group, and in only 38.3% of the control group. It was noted after three days that the white blood cell count had already increased over $4 \times 10^9/L$ in 49.6% of the warming needling group and 42.5% of the moxibustion group, but only 2.9% in the control group. The acupoints used in this study were: Zusanli (ST 36), Sanyinjiao (SP 6), Neiguan (PC 6),

Yinlingquan (SP 9), Guanyuan (CV 4), Qihai (CV 6) and Xuehai (SP 10) for warming needling; and Dazhui (GV 14), Geshu (BL 17), Pishu (BL 20), Weishu (BL 21), and Shenshu (BL 23) for moxa cone moxibustion.

2. Increasing Sensitivity to Chemotherapy and Radiotherapy

Increasing sensitivity to chemotherapy and radiotherapy has dual implications: either to promote original efficacy with the routine dosage, or to obtain similar effect with a smaller dose. Both are designed to improve the results of chemotherapy and radiotherapy.

All the herbal therapies mentioned above may serve this purpose, but those which strengthen body resistance are most advantageous. Both chemotherapy and radiotherapy are aggressive treatments which kill tumor cells and at the same time harm normal cells. Body resistance is thus further impaired. From the traditional medical point of view, protection of body resistance is of crucial importance with any aggressive treatment. It is aimed not only at amelioration of adverse effects, but also at promoting therapeutic effects.

The advantageous effect of body-resistance-strengthening therapy has been proven repeatedly in clinical investigation; many herbal formulae can be used to this end. The following is a well-known traditional formula called *Si Junzi Tang* (SJT; Decoction of Four Noble Ingredients). It consists of: Radix Ginseng (ginseng) or Radix Codonopsis Pilosulae (pilose asiabell root), Poria (poria), Rhizoma Atractylodis Macrocephalae (white atractylodes rhizome), and Radix Glycyrrhizae Praeparata (prepared licorice).

Primary carcinoma of the liver has been considered insensitive to radiotherapy. Tumor Hospital of Shanghai Medical University studied the combined use of SJT with radiotherapy from 1980 to 1991 in 228 cases of intermediate liver carcinoma. The rate of survival over five years was 42.97% and the median survival 53.4 months in the combined treatment group, while in the group treated with radiotherapy and other medicines not related to SJT, the rate of survival over five years was 14.48% and the median survival 11.1 months. This striking difference indicates that SJT increases the sensitivity of primary liver carcinoma to radiotherapy. It was also noted that those receiving SJT had almost no adverse response to the radiotherapy. About half the patients had a good appetite, and one-third even gained weight during the period of radiotherapy. Animal experiments have also confirmed these results. Nude mice implanted with human liver carcinoma cells were treated with three different schemes: one group with radiotherapy alone, another group with SJT alone, and the third group with radiotherapy and SJT. Results showed control of the tumor growth and the longest survival in the third group.

Herbs used to remove blood stasis are also effective. Some argue against using blood-stasis-removing therapy as the sole form of treatment for cancer, for though improvement of local blood circulation facilitates the host's resistance against tumor on the one hand, there is also an increased risk of tumor metastasis. When used in conjunction with chemotherapy, however, it increases sensitivity by improving local blood circulation, which allows the cytotoxic agent access to the tumor. Danger of tumor metastasis is minimized by the existence of a cytotoxic agent in the blood. Radix Salviae Miltiorrhizae (red sage root), that very drug which has been shown to promote cancer metastasis in animals, works as such in combination with chemotherapy. Radix Salviae Miltiorrhizae and a COP schedule of chemotherapy (administration of cyclophosphamide, oncovin and prednisolone) has been shown to have a synergic effect in the treatment of malignant lymphoma: there is longer clinical remission and more marked regression of enlarged lymph nodes than those treated with COP schedule alone.

The question of whether or not to use toxic-heat-eliminating therapy in combination with chemotherapy and radiotherapy is rather complicated. Theoretically, long-term use of these drugs will further deteriorate body resistance, but some do have a positive effect when used in this way, probably due to the multiplicity of their pharmacological actions.

Much research is being conducted on the use of herbal medication to reduce toxicity of chemotherapy and radiotherapy and enhance sensitivity to these therapies. The present trend is to use a combination of the various categories, particularly those which strengthen body resistance and remove blood stasis.

Herbal Medicines in the Prevention of Cancer

Another interesting question is whether herbal medication can be used to prevent cancer, which is the result of the prolonged action of carcinogenic factors in a body with lowered resistance. Approaches to prevention of cancer are thus elimination of the carcinogenic factors and reinforcement of body resistance. Many of the tonics mentioned in Chapter IV are likely to help prevent cancer.

Among the pathogenetic factors apt to result in the growth of cancer, some chronic inflammatory diseases should be taken as precancerous lesions which will cause epithelial cell proliferation and malignant change over time. Treatment of these precancerous diseases is important in the prevention of cancer, but such a discussion (such as treatment of chronic atrophic gastritis for the prevention of stomach cancer, or treatment of chronic hepatitis for the prevention of liver cancer) is beyond the scope of this chapter. However, treatment of esophageal epithelial hyperplasia in the high-risk areas of esophageal carcinoma should not be omitted, because this is one treatment aimed solely at cancer prevention.

Institute of Materia Medica, China Academy of Traditional Chinese Medicine, studied the use of *Liuwei Dihuang Wan* (LDW; Pill of Six Ingredients with Rehmannia) in the prevention of esophageal carcinoma. Like SJT mentioned above, LDW is also a well-known herbal formula composed of tonics. The ingredients are: Radix Rehmanniae Praeparata (prepared rehmannia root), Fructus Corni (dogwood fruit), Rhizoma Dioscoreae (Chinese yam), Rhizoma Alismatis (alismatis rhizome), Poria (poria) and Cortex Moutan Radicis (moutan bark). It works to strengthen body resistance, but with a different mechanism from that of SJT. SJT, a preparation of *qi* tonics, strengthens the functional processes, including that of body resistance against cancer and other diseases; LDW, a preparation of *yin* tonics, replenishes the essential materials needed for the body resistance. Modern research has shown that both enhance the immune function when it is low, but they probably act on different links: SJT effects cellular immunity to promote phagocytosis, while LDW works on humoral immunity to prolong the presence of circulating antibodies. Their other actions are to improve digestion and assimilation (SJT) and regulate the sexual endocrine function (LDW).

LDW has been shown to inhibit the occurrence of experimentally induced progastric squamous carcinoma in mice. It was administered in 92 cases of esophageal hyperplasia where esophageal carcinoma prevailed. After one year, only two cases experienced cancerization, the epithelial hyperplasia remained the same in eight and improved or returned to normal in 82; while in the control group of 89 with esophageal hyperplasia which received no LDW, cancerization occurred in 11 cases, and hyperplasia remained the same in 23 and improved in 55. This statistical difference indicates the great effect of LDW in prevention of esophageal carcinoma.

Some anti-cancer herbs can also be used for prevention. Quite a few of the toxic-heat-eliminating herbs have been found to have cancer-inhibiting effect. When used as the sole treatment for cancer, their effect is not always satisfactory, probably because they are not potent enough to kill tumor cells when a tumor already exists. But most anti-cancer herbs have low toxicity levels. In addition, they may have actions other than inhibition of the nucleic acid metabolism of the tumor cells. They are thus useful for prevention.

A tablet preparation containing Radix Sophorae Subprostratae (subprostrate sophora root), Herba Patriniae (patrinia herb) and other toxic-heat-eliminating herbs have been shown to prevent experimental progastric squamous carcinoma in mice. Of 72 cases of serious esophageal hyperplasia, improvement was found in 61.8% (the natural improvement rate was only 29.8%, as revealed in the control group of 215 which received nothing).

From the above, it can be seen that traditional Chinese medicine has been used to treat cancer throughout history. The strategy of strengthening body resistance to the disease merits special attention, for it provides a rational approach quite different from that of Western medicine. The use of herbal medication to minimize toxic and side effects and enhance the therapeutic effect of chemotherapy and radiotherapy is also worth note, particularly as these therapies are undergoing rapid expansion, and new forms of treatment are being developed.

CHAPTER VII
ACUPUNCTURE AND MOXIBUSTION

Acupuncture and moxibustion have been applied as therapeutic techniques in China for more than 2,000 years. Because of their many indications, minimal side effects, low cost and rapid therapeutic effect, these ancient healing arts have remained popular for ages. Recent research has not only confirmed their effectiveness, but has also provided modern scientific explanations for why they work.

Meridians and Acupuncture Points

The theoretical basis of acupuncture and moxibustion is the theory of the meridians. According to this theory, there is a system of meridians (also called channels) in the body through which *qi* (vital energy) and blood circulate, and by which internal organs are coordinated and connected with superficial organs and tissues, creating an integral whole. There are certain points along the superficial part of the meridians reached by *qi* of the visceral organs. Acupuncturists use these points, called acupuncture points or acupoints; they are the places where the body surface is connected with the visceral organs. When one is ill, the flow of *qi* and blood can be regulated by stimulating certain points of the body surface through needling or moxibustion; illness of the associated internal organs can thus be cured.

The cardinal conduits of vital energy and blood are called meridians, and the branches of the meridians, collaterals. Meridians are divided into regular meridians and extra meridians. The 12 pairs of regular meridians constitute most of the meridian system. There are eight extra meridians. The 12 regular meridians plus the two extra meridians, one running along the midline of the abdomen and chest, and the other along the midline of the back, are the 14 meridians.

The 12 meridians are symmetrically distributed over both sides of the body, and run respectively through the medial or lateral side of each limb. Each meridian pertains to one visceral organ and is thus named. The English names of the 12 meridians and the alphabetic codes recommended by the World Health Organization are listed as follows:

The Lung Meridian (LU), Pericardium Meridian (PC) and Heart Meridian (HT) run through the anterior aspect, midline and posterior aspect of the anterior side of the upper limbs from the chest to the hands. They are collectively called the Three *Yin* Meridians of the Hand.

The Large Intestine Meridian (LI), Triple Energizer Meridian (TE) and Small Intestine Meridian (SI) run through the anterior aspect, midline and posterior aspect of the medial side of the upper limbs from the hands to the head. They are collectively called the Three *Yang* Meridians of the Hand.

The Spleen Meridian (SP), Liver Meridian (LR) and Kidney Meridian (KI) run respectively through the anterior aspect, midline and posterior aspect of the medial side of the lower limbs from the feet to the abdomen and the chest. They are collectively called the Three *Yin* Meridians of the Foot.

The Stomach Meridian (ST), Gallbladder Meridian (GB) and Bladder Meridian (BL) run from the head through the trunk to the feet along the anterior aspect, midline and posterior aspect of the lateral side of the lower limbs. They are collectively called the Three *Yang* Meridians of the Foot.

The extra meridian running along the midline of the abdomen and chest upward to the lower lip is called the Conception Vessel (CV).

The extra meridian running along the midline of the back upward to the top of the head and then downward to the middle of the face is called the Governor Vessel (GV).

Three hundren and sixty-one acupuncture points have been identified along the 14 meridians. The standard nomenclature of these points consists of the Chinese phonetic (*pinyin*) name followed by the alphanumeric code in parenthesis. Apart from these, there are a number of acupuncture points with specific therapeutic properties not on the 14 meridians; they are called extraordinary points.

Each acupuncture point has its own therapeutic action. For example, the point Hegu (LI 4), located between the first and second metacarpal bones, can sedate pain in the head and mouth. It is indicated for headache, toothache and sore throat. The point Shenmen (HT 7), located on the medial end of the transverse crease of the wrist, can induce tranquilization. It is indicated for insomnia. Yanglingquan (GB 34), located at the lateral aspect of the knee-joint, in the depression anterior and inferior to the head of the fibula, is indicated in the treatment of gallbladder diseases, shoulder pain and stiff neck; Yinlingquan (SP 9), located in the depression on the lower border of the medial condyle of the tibia, is indicated in the treatment of retention or incontinence of urine, and seminal emission.

Technique and Methods

In ordinary clinics, acupuncture is performed with thin filiform needles. The needles are made of stainless steel and vary in length (from 1 cm to 15 cm) and in diameter (from 0.27 mm to 0.46 mm). The needle is selected according to the depth of insertion required. For instance, needling a point on the buttock usually requires a long thick needle, while a point on the scalp will require a short thin needle.

After local sterilization, the needles are inserted perpendicularly or obliquely at the points to the required depth. If the point is correctly located and the required depth reached, the patient will usually experience a feeling of soreness, heaviness, numbness and distention. This acupuncture sensation indicates successful application. The manipulator will simultaneously feel a tightness in the needle. The acupuncture sensation may be transmitted along a certain path; when pointed out by the patient, it is usually consistent with the theoretical path of the meridian.

After the needle is inserted, it may be manipulated according to the specifications of treatment for the disease. Generally speaking, illnesses can be divided into three categories. The first two are those with deficiency or excess syndrome. Deficiency syndrome is characterized by diminished body function, while excess syndrome refers to excess of pathogenic factors accompanied by physical hyperfunctioning. In the third category are those not so distinct or jumbled cases with both deficiency of body function and excess of pathogenic factors. Needle manipulations are also divided into three categories: reinforcement, reduction and uniform reinforcement-reduction. Reinforcement means to activate and restore hypofunction to normal. Reduction means to expel pathogenic factors and restore hyperfunction to normal. The needles are usually twirled or "lift-thrust" at the specified point. When the twirling method is used, the needle is twisted slowly and rotated in small circles for reinforcement; it is twisted quickly and rotated in large circles for reduction. When the lift-thrust method is used, reinforcement and reduction can be attained by varying the force of lifting and thrusting the needle. Uniform reinforcement-reduction is attained by lifting and thrusting or twisting and twirling the needle evenly with moderate force. Recent research indicates that mild manipulation works to reinforce because it induces excitation; strong manipulation works to reduce because it induces inhibition; and moderate manipulation works to reinforce-reduce because it induces modulation. The needles are usually left *in situ* for 15-30 minutes or longer. During this time, reinforcing or reducing manipulations may be repeated.

Needling may also be activated by pulsatile electrical stimulation. This procedure is called electro-acupuncture. Reinforcing and reducing manipulations can be attained by varying frequency and voltage.

An acupuncture-like effect can be obtained by deep finger pressure, or acupressure. In acupressure treatment, the points are pressed with the thumb, tip of the middle finger or edge of the finger nail. For example, pressing Renzhong (GV 26), located between the upper and middle third of the philtrum, may stop one from fainting; pressing Hegu (LI 4), located half way along the line between the first and second metacarpal bones and the middle of the web between the thumb and index finger, may stop toothache and arrest an attack of asthma.

Other approaches to stimulation of acupuncture points include use of ultrasound and lasers.

Ear-acupuncture (or auriculo-acupuncture) is a derivative of ordinary acupuncture. In auriculo-acupuncture, ear needles are used at sensitive points in corresponding regions of the ear. The needles are usually like a thumb-nail or wheat-grain in shape and fixed with adhesive plaster after insertion. The ear needles may be replaced by vaccaria seeds to be pressed by the patient at regular intervals after leaving the doctor's office.

Moxibustion is often used in combination with acupuncture, but it may also be performed separately. The main difference between moxibustion and acupuncture is that the former applies heat instead of mechanical stimulus to the point. It is indicated chiefly for deficiency syndromes with cold manifestations such as pain aggravated by cold. Moxa wool, made of dry moxa leaves (Artemisia vulgaris) ground into a cotton-like substance, is shaped into a moxa stick about 20 cm long and 1.4 cm in diameter. An ignited moxa stick is held about an inch from the patient's skin, warming the point until it reddens or it is held nearer to the skin and moved up and down so as to apply more heat to the point. A single treatment of moxibustion usually lasts 10-15 minutes.

Other methods, such as direct and indirect moxibustion with moxa cone, are still used. In direct and indirect moxibustion, the moxa wool is shaped into a cone, the diameter at the base 0.4-0.7 cm and the height 0.3-1.0 cm. Direct moxibustion is performed by placing the moxa cone directly on the point and then igniting it. Indirect moxibustion, also called partition moxibustion, uses a layer of herb paste or slice of ginger, garlic or aconite between the skin and the smoldering moxa cone. The ignited cone should generally be removed and replaced with a new one whenever the patient feels pain; about three-seven cones are necessary for a single treatment.

Needle-warming moxibustion combines needling and moxibustion by attaching a moxa stub (about 2 cm long) to an inserted needle. Usually one-three stubs are burned during the treatment. This method enhances the effects of needling and is often used to treat chronic rheumatism and rheumatoid arthritis.

Indications and Contraindications

Acupuncture is a non-specific therapy which aims to regulate various body functions. It may be used clinically as the primary treatment or as an adjunct for relieving certain symptoms. In 1979 the World Health Organization formulated a list of 43 diseases that can be treated by acupuncture. Recently, however, it has been reported effective for about 250 kinds of diseases. Its special therapeutic effect has been shown to work with diseases refractory to Western treatment: immune diseases, drug addictions, psychogenic diseases and functional disorders. The indications in Chinese acupuncture textbooks are usually listed as follows:

(1) Medical diseases: Common cold, influenza, bronchitis, bronchial asthma, epigastric pain, vomiting, hiccup, abdominal pain, diarrhea, dysentery, abdominal distention, constipation, hypertension, cardiac palpitation, malaria, arthritis.

(2) Surgical and orthopedic disorders: Lumbar pain, shoulder pain, elbow pain, sprain, strained neck, acute appendicitis,

cholelithiasis, mastitis, simple goiter, prolapse of rectum.

(3) Gynecological and obstetrical disorders: Irregular menstruation, dysmenorrhea, amenorrhea, pelvic inflammation, prolapse of uterus, morning sickness, malposition of fetus, prolonged labor, lactation deficiency.

(4) Pediatric diseases: Whooping cough, infantile malnutrition, acute infantile convulsion, chronic infantile convulsion, paralysis due to poliomyelitis.

(5) Urogenital disorders: Enuresis, retention of urine, seminal emission, impotence, infections of the urinary tract.

(6) Nervous and mental disorders: Apoplexy, paraplegia, epilepsy, headache, trigeminal neuralgia, facial paralysis, sciatica, multiple neuritis, neurasthenia, hysteria, depression, schizophrenia.

(7) Diseases of the sense organs and neighboring structures: Acute conjunctivitis, myopia, atrophy of optic nerve, tonsillitis, pharyngitis, chronic rhinitis, chronic sinusitis, epistaxis, toothache, tinnitus, deafness.

It should be noted that this list of indications is based on clinical experience. In recent years, controlled clinical research has shown further evidence of the efficacy of acupuncture and its related therapies. The following are some examples.

Examples of Acupuncture Treatment of Common Diseases

Cerebral Infarction

Cerebral infarction with hemiplegia is one of the most common indications of acupuncture treatment. However, since the patients often improve naturally, it is difficult to assess the therapeutic effect in uncontrolled clinical studies. Recently, a comparative study was carried out by Beijing College of Acupuncture-Moxibustion and Orthopedics-Traumatology. Sixty-three patients suffering from cerebral infarction (as diagnosed by CT scanning and lumbar puncture) were divided into two groups: 32 were treated with acupuncture, and 31 with Calan, a drug manufactured by Takeda Co. commonly prescribed for cerebral infarction. Standards stipulated by the All-China Association of Traditional Chinese Medicine were used to assess the effect of treatment.

After six weeks, 20 (62.5%) of the acupuncture group were basically cured and 4 (12.5%) markedly improved, for a total effective rate of 75%; 8 (25.8%) of the Calan group were basically cured and 5 (16.1%) markedly improved, for a total effective rate of 42%. Hemorheological studies carried out on these patients showed marked difference in rheological indices compared with healthy individuals before treatment: high blood platelet aggregation, blood specific viscosity, and hematocrit. These indices were lowered after treatment in both groups; the authors believe that acupuncture treatment ameliorates cerebral ischemia and hastens recovery of paralytic limbs due to improvement of blood rheology.

In the acupuncture treatment, Jianyu (LI 15), Quchi (LI 11), Hegu (LI 4), Huantiao (GB 30), Yanglingquan (GB 34) and Guangming (GB 37) are main points for needling with lifting-thrusting manipulation. Reduction is used when the paralysis is spastic and reinforcement when the paralysis is flaccid. Transmission of sensation to the distal end of the limb or muscular twitching of the limb is required. The needling should be performed daily for six weeks.

Depression

From 1981 to 1984, the Institute of Mental Health, Beijing Medical University studied the effect of electro-acupuncture treatment on depression. Antidepressant amitriptyline was used as the control drug. Preliminary observation had shown that electro-acupuncture had a similar effect as the amitriptyline but with fewer side effects. In order to verify the clinical effect of electro-acupuncture in the treatment of depression, ten institutes and hospitals specializing in mental disease collaborated on a study of 241 patients. Each institution divided the patients into two groups: 133 received electro-acupuncture treatment and 108 were given amitriptyline. Hamilton's Depression Rating Scale was used to assess the therapeutic effects. After treatment, the scores in the electro-acupuncture group were reduced from 35.3 ± 0.7 to 8.3 ± 0.7; in the amitriptyline group they were reduced from 35.5 ± 0.8 to 10.4 ± 1.1. There was no significant difference between the two groups. Further analysis showed that electro-acupuncture had a similar therapeutic effect as amitriptyline on manic-depressives, but a better effect on reactive depressives. As for individual syndromes, electro-acupuncture had a similar effect on psychomotor retardation, sleep disorders and hopelessness as amitriptyline, but a better effect on anxiety and cognition disturbance. Asberger's Side Effect Scale of Antidepressants indicated that those treated with amitriptyline experienced a higher rate of cardiovascular, extrapyramidal and anticholinergic reaction than those treated with electro-acupuncture. Biochemical and electro-physiological examinations performed on 89 of the patients suggested varying therapeutic mechanisms between electro-acupuncture and amitriptyline.

Correction of Abnormal Fetal Position by Auriculo-acupressure

It has been shown repeatedly that abnormal fetal position, a common cause of difficult labor, can be corrected by moxibustion. In a controlled clinical study by a hospital in Jiangsu Province, of 150 cases of abnormal fetal position in the third trimester, 110 were treated with auriculo-acupressure and 40 with knee-chest position. For auriculo-acupressure, the points on one ear were detected with an acupuncture needle, the skin sterilized with 75% alcohol, and vaccaria seeds taped over the points with adhesive plaster. The patient was asked to press and knead the seeds every day before breakfast, lunch and supper, five minutes each time. After four days the patient was re-examined. If the fetal position was still abnormal, similar therapy was applied to the other ear with new seeds. In the control group, knee-chest position was adopted twice a day for 10-15 minutes in the morning and evening. After one week, if the fetal position was still abnormal, another course of treatment was advised. If the fetal position turned to normal after one-four courses of auriculo-acupressure or one-two courses of knee-chest position as confirmed by obstetrical examination (including ultrasonic examination), the treatment was considered as a success. The success rate was 84.5% in the auriculo-acupressure group, and 67.5% in the control group. The difference was even more marked in those with a gestation period over 33 weeks: 77.5% in the auriculo-acupressure group vs. 35.7% in the control group. In the auriculo-acupressure group, no adverse effects were observed in either the patient or the fetus. In all cases, fetal movements were counted for an hour in the morning, at noon and in the evening. They were found to have increased in most cases during auriculo-acupressure, suggesting that the fetal position was corrected through stimulation of the points.

Chemotherapy-induced Leukopenia

Decrease of white blood cells is a common side effect of chemotherapy which may in some cases cause interruption and failure of the therapy. Acupuncture had been used to treat leukopenia of various causes with success. The study made by Henan Tumor Hospital and other collaborating institutions showing evidence of the therapeutic effect of acupuncture-moxibustion in the treatment of chemotherapy-induced leukopenia has already been discussed in Chapter VI.

Besides these controlled clinical studies, laboratory data may also give evidence of the therapeutic effects of acupuncture treatment. The following are examples where, though controlled tests are difficult to carry out, the results obtained in the biochemical assays are convincing.

Male Infertility

Fujian Institute of Traditional Chinese Medicine reported a series of 160 cases of oligospermia with a history of infertility for at least one year. The results of treatment with acupuncture and indirect moxibustion were satisfactory: oligospermia was cured in 78.1% of the cases, and 85.0% of the wives of those cured became pregnant. Another group of 32 patients with oligospermia showed similar results: 28 (87.5%) were cured, as the sperm count increased to more than 6 x 10^7/ml with normal sperm motility and morphology; 23 (82.1%) of the wives of those cured became pregnant after treatment. Blood chorionic gonadotropin (HCG) and testosterone (T) levels were determined by radio-immunoassay to investigate the change in secretion of hormones after acupuncture-moxibustion treatment. In comparison with the results obtained from a group of 32 fertile men, both blood HCG and T levels were lower in the infertility cases. After 15 days of acupuncture and indirect ginger moxibustion treatment, both blood HCG and T had risen to the levels of those in the fertile group.

The treatment adopted was a combination of acupuncture and indirect ginger moxibustion. Acupuncture was performed with reinforcing twisting manipulation until acupuncture sensation was experienced; indirect ginger moxibustion with three cones was then applied at each point. Two groups of acupoints were selected. Group I: Dahe (KI 12), Qugu (CV 2) and Sanyinjiao (SP 6) for acupuncture, and Guanyuan (CV 4) and Zhongji (CV 3) for moxibustion. Group II: Baliao (BL 31-34) and Shenshu (BL 23) for acupuncture, and Shenshu (BL 23) and Mingmen (GV 4) for moxibustion. These two groups were used alternately every other day.

Obesity

Acupuncture is believed to be an effective means to reduce body weight in obese individuals, but since food intake is the primary cause of simple obesity, it is difficult to perform a controlled study which rules out this factor. A report from Nanjing College of Traditional Chinese Medicine provides more evidence about the anti-obesity effect of acupuncture. It was found that after a one-month course of treatment there was a reduction in body weight of an average of 3.4 kg, with corresponding reduction in chest, waist, hip and thigh measurements. Blood lipid analysis also showed a decrease of serum triglyceride, total cholesterol, low density lipoprotein-cholesterol and very low density lipoprotein-cholesterol; and an increase of high density lipoprotein-cholesterol. Such changes are beneficial for prevention of atherosclerosis. Plasma adrenocorticotropic hormone (ACTH) and saliva cortisol (CS) assay revealed that both plasma ACTH and saliva CS, which were lower than normal before treatment, increased thereafter. These changes are related to the therapeutic effects: There was a marked rise of plasma ACTH and saliva CS after treatment in those cases which lost the most weight, a moderate rise of these indices in those which lost a moderate amount, and no rise in those where there was no change of body weight. The authors' conclusion is that acupuncture works on obesity by enhancing the function of the hypothalamus-pituitary-adrenal system.

The acupuncture method adopted was a combination of ordinary acupuncture and ear acupuncture; the acupoints were selected according to traditional differentiation of symptom-complexes. Recent reports have also shown that auriculo-acupressure may also achieve a similar effect in reducing body weight with simple obesity.

Another way to confirm the therapeutic effect of acupuncture is through treatment of experimental models. Since most factors in animal experiments can be strictly controlled, the results are usually reliable as supplementary evidence. This is illustrated in the following example.

Bronchial Asthma

Bronchial asthma is a common allergic disease with repeated paroxysmal attacks. Although there are a variety of antiasthmatic drugs available for inducing remission, there are often side effects with prolonged use. Acupuncture has been widely used to treat bronchial asthma, either for immediate remission or over the long term. Most of the points used are distributed along the lung and large intestine meridians of the arms, as well as some points on the back. The Second Municipal Hospital in Kaifeng has reported immediate effect of acupuncture treatment for relieving asthmatic attacks. They selected bilateral Kongzui (LU 6) and Yuji (LU 10) points for ordinary needling with reducing manipulation followed by electric continuous-wave stimulation at 160 Hz and moderate intensity. Kongzui (LU 6) is located on the anterior aspect of the forearm, between the proximal 5/12 and distal 7/12 of the line joining Taiyuan (LU 9) in the depression distal to the styloid process of the radius above the wrist and Chize (LU 5) on the transverse cubital crease at the lateral border of the biceps. Yuji (LU 10) is located at the midpoint of the border of the thenar eminence. Of the 192 cases studied, clinical remission was achieved in 59 cases and marked improvement in 85 cases within ten minutes; 75% were thus totally or essentially relieved of asthmatic attack. A comparative clinical study showed that acupuncture at Kongzui (LU 6) had more rapid and long-lasting anti-asthmatic effect than oral aminophylline. Experiments on guinea pigs demonstrated the curative effect of acupuncture at Kongzui (LU 6) on asthma induced by histamine. Needling at Yuji (LU 10) in the guinea pigs enhanced the pulmonary content of cAMP and raised the value of cAMP/cGMP ratio. These changes are consistent with the relief of bronchial contraction.

Besides its application to treating various diseases, acupuncture can also be used for the following purposes: anti-aging treatment, rehabilitation, cosmetology, and abstinence from smoking and drug addictions.

The contraindications of acupuncture include pregnancy (when associated with diseases otherwise amenable to acupuncture), needling of tumor sites, skin infections, presence of a cardiac pacemaker, and coexisting hemorrhagic diathesis. There are risks attendant to needle insertion in the body in areas where vital structures, such as arteries, lungs, liver, spleen and intestines, could inadvertently be punctured. Fainting, due to nervousness, weakness, fatigue, hunger, improper posture of the patient or excessively strong stimulation, may also occur. Rest is the best remedy, though emergency treatment is occasionally required.

Therapeutic Mechanism

Acupuncture is effective for both inducing and checking sweating, for relieving both diarrhea and constipation, for treating both retention of urine and enuresis. Recent clinical and experimental studies indicate that the therapeutic effects of acupuncture can be attributed to regulation of body functions; even its analgesic effect can be taken as a regulatory action. However, since the mechanism of acupuncture analgesia has been extensively studied, it will be discussed separately.

How does acupuncture produce an excitatory effect in some cases but inhibitory effects in others? There are three factors to consider: the functional state of the patient, the acupuncture points selected, and the kind of stimulus given.

1. Functional State of the Patient

The functional state of the patient is the most important factor. For example, it has been repeatedly confirmed that needling with the same intensity at the same acupoint or group of acupoints attenuates gastrointestinal peristalsis if in a hyperactive state, and enhances gastrointestinal peristalsis if in a hypoactive state. Further, an excitatory effect is produced when the central nervous system is in a state of inhibition, and an inhibitory effect when it is in a state of excitation; a hypotensive effect in a state of hypertension and a hypertensive effect in a state of hypotension; an immuno-enhancing effect in a state of decreased immune function, and an immuno-inhibiting effect in a state of abnormally increased immune functions; a diuretic effect in a state of oliguria induced by pitressin, and an antidiuretic effect in a state of polyuria induced by hypertonic glucose injection.

In some other instances, though different functional states may not produce entirely different or opposite effects, they may greatly influence the result. For example, the analgesic effect of acupuncture varies with each patient. Acupuncture analgesia usually works well with patients with *yang*-deficiency as manifested by pale complexion, quiescence, aversion to cold, cold limbs, pale tongue with whitish coating, and slow pulse; it is often less satisfactory in patients with *yin*-deficiency as manifested by flushing face or malar flush, irritability, aversion to heat, heat sensation in the palm and soles, reddened tongue with scanty coating or yellowish coating, and rapid pulse.

2. Intensity of Stimulation

The close relationship between the functional state of the patient and the effect of acupuncture does not exclude the other two factors. Proper manipulation with appropriate intensity and duration of stimulation usually gives the desired effect, whereas too strong or too weak a stimulus produces little or no effect. Such a case has been illustrated through the preventive treatment of leukopenia with acupuncture in patients with mammary cancer who were receiving chemotherapy after surgical operation. Reinforcing manipulation with weak stimulation gave the best results: the white blood cell count began to drop after three weeks of chemotherapy. In the group treated by reducing manipulation with strong stimulation, the white blood cell count began to drop after only two weeks of chemotherapy. The group which received no preventive treatment was the worst off: the white blood cell count dropped the very first week of chemotherapy. From this study we can see the effect of acupuncture on leukopenia prevention during chemotherapy, and how its efficacy varies with different intensities of stimulation.

Another question is whether stimuli of different intensity can exert the opposite effect. Such a result has been found in animal experiments: weak stimulation causes dilatation of blood vessels and increased intestinal movements, while strong stimulation causes constriction of blood vessels and inhibition of intestinal movements. The same has been observed in normal human subjects, but when morbid conditions prevail, the opposite effect seldom occurs. There have been very few reports showing opposite response during application of strong and weak stimulation. A self-controlled study of arthritis patients showed dilatation of blood vessels during weak stimulation and constriction of blood vessels during strong stimulation as demonstrated by volume of blood flow.

3. Selection of Acupoints

The therapeutic effect of acupuncture is naturally related to the acupoints selected for treatment. First of all, in most instances only the acupoints should be needled to produce therapeutic effect. This raises a question about the peculiarities of these acupoints. Morphological studies of cutanenous and subcutaneous tissues show differences between tissues at the acupoint site and those elsewhere on the body surface. Most authors agree that the acupoint site is rich with nerve endings. The possibility of a special structure at the acupoint site is still under investigation.

Biophysical features of the acupoints are more pronounced. The low electrical resistance of the skin at the acupoint site has been confirmed. It is interesting to note that disease may lead to changes of the skin electrical resistance at the corresponding acupoints. For example, acute gastric disorders may result in further lowering of skin resistance at the acupoints along the Stomach Meridian. Similar changes may also be brought about at the ear points. The electrical resistance of ear points Zigong (Uterus), Luanchao (Ovary) and Neifenmi (Endocrine) varies with the menstrual cycle: it is lower during menstration and ovulation than other times of the month.

Low electrical resistance at certain sites corresponding to acupoints also exists in animals. It helps locate the acupoints when conducting animal experiments. There is, however, some argument about the relationship between points with low resistance and the acupoints. Most acupoints exhibit low resistance, but not all points with low resistance are consistent with the location of recognized acupoints. Even more debatable is why electrical resistance is lower at the acupoint sites. Though many hypotheses have been proposed, none has yet been proven. Probably the most convincing evidence is to be found by looking at the clinical features.

Tenderness, induration and biophysical changes occur frequently at the sites of corresponding acupoints. It was reported that with liver disease, there was tenderness in 95% of the cases at Ganshu (BL 18; a point on the back below the spinous process of the ninth thoracic vertebra about 1.5 *cun** lateral to the posterior midline); there was

---

* One method used in acupuncture therapy for locating points is finger measurement. When the middle finger is flexed, the distance between the medial ends of the two interphalangeal creases of the patient's middle finger is taken as one *cun*.

such tenderness in only 24% of the cases at Pishu (BL 20, a point located the back below the spinous process of the 11th vertebra 1.5 *cun* lateral to the posterior midline). In patients with infection of the biliary tract and gall stone, tenderness was found in 77% of the cases at Tianzong (SI 11, a point located in the depression at the center of the infrascapular fossa); healthy individuals and patients with peptic ulcer, hemorrhoids or periarthritis of the shoulder, exhibited no such tenderness.

Tender points may thus provide clues to the location of new acupoints. Discovery of Lanwei (Appendix, EX-LE 7), a point in the upper part of the anterior surface of the leg, five *cun* below the depression lateral to the patella and its ligament and one finger-breadth lateral to the anterior crest of the tibia, is one such example. This point is widely used for acupuncture treatment of appendicitis.

Needling of different acupoints show different results. This is particularly true for acupoints along the various meridians. Some acupoints are specifically effective in treating certain diseases. A comparative study of needling at Neiguan (PC 6) and Sanyinjiao (SP 6) in patients with coronary heart disease showed the following difference: With Neiguan (PC 6), a specific point for treating heart disease, there was marked improvement of the left ventricular function as revealed by shortened preejection and isovolumetric contraction phases. Needling at Sanyinjiao (SP 6), however, brought about no such changes.

In another study of 70 cases of stomach disease with epigastric pain patients were divided into two groups: 40 were treated with acupuncture at the points Pishu (BL 20) and Weishu (BL 21), as routinely selected for stomach problems, and 30 were treated with acupuncture at Dachangshu (BL 25) and Qihaishu (BL 24), which are ordinarily used for diseases of the large intestine and lumbago but not for the stomach. After 20 minutes most patients in the first group felt better and treatment was conducted, but only five in the second group experienced alleviation from pain. The remaining 25 were then treated with Pishu (BL 20) and Weishu (BL 21). Rate of effectiveness with Pishu (BL 20) and Weishu (BL 21) was 93.8% and that with other two irrelevant acupoints was 16.7%. The above four acupoints are all located along the same meridian which runs longitudinally down the back at slightly different horizontal levels. The difference in therapeutic effect indicates the specific actions of these acupoints.

As mentioned above, acupuncture depends primarily upon three factors: the functional state of the patient, the acupoints selected and the manipulation (pattern and intensity of stimulation). An experienced acupuncturist can select the most proper acupoints and best pattern and intensity of stimulation for the best results.

Acupuncture to Combat Pain

Pain is the most common symptom of disease. About half the patients who visit a physician complain of pain. Although the correct treatment of disease alleviates pain, the patient may first need relief in this regard at the onset; with some uncontrolled pain continues to be a major problem.

Relief of pain is the most prominent therapeutic effect of acupuncture and probably one of the most important reasons why this unique treatment has won recognition throughout the world. Acupuncture analgesia can be used for any condition associated with pain, so long as the needling is not substituted for other necessary treatment. The best example of acupuncture analgesia is its use in place of anesthesia for surgical operations.

I. Brief History of the Development of "Acupuncture Anesthesia"

Acupuncture analgesia was first used in cases of tonsillectomy in Shanghai First Municipal Hospital in 1958. A report on 74 patients who underwent the operation under acupuncture analgesia was published in *Shanghai Journal of Traditional Medicine* in January 1959. During those years acupuncture analgesia was used at Xi'an Fourth Municipal Hospital in the fields of gynecology, dentistry, ophthalmology and general surgery. Of 875 patients operated on under "acupuncture anesthesia," no pain was felt by 630 (72.0%) and mild pain by 195 (22.3%). Fifty patients (5.6%) experienced pain. "Acupuncture anesthesia" has since spread all over China. In June 1979, the First National Symposium on Acupuncture-Moxibustion and Acupuncture Anesthesia was held in Beijing. One hundred and forty-nine of the participants came from 32 countries and areas abroad. Since 1979 research on "acupuncture anesthesia" has been focused on improvement of its anesthetic effect with supplementary anesthetic or analgesic drugs and official approval of its indications.

The criteria for assessing anesthetic effect were stipulated in 1981 as follows: Excellent — with minimal anesthetic or analgesic drug, the patient experiences no pain or discomfort during the operation; Good — with less than one-third the dosage used in drug anesthesia, the patient basically experiences no pain or discomfort during the operation. Failure — the acupuncture anesthesia requires supplementary anesthetic or has to be replaced by drug anesthesia.

Accord ing to the above, application of "acupuncture anesthesia" has been officially approved for a number of operations: such as thyroidectomy, operations on the anterior cranium and brain, pneumectory, subtotal gastrectomy, abdominal ligation of fallopian tubes, and abdominal hysterectomy.

II. Advantages and Disadvantages of "Acupuncture Anesthesia"

"Acupuncture anesthesia" is probably a misnomer if anesthesia is defined as inducing loss of sensation. Acupuncture can only raise one's pain threshold; it cannot induce loss of sensation. Therefore, as a kind of anesthesia, acupuncture has its disadvantages: incomplete extirpation of pain, insufficient muscular relaxation and visceral traction response. Use of acupuncture analgesia in operation is nonetheless worthy of recommendation not only out of academic interest but also for practical use. It has the following advantages over drug anesthesia:

1) It is safe. Of the several million patients in China who have undergone operation under "acupuncture anesthesia," not a single one has died of this cause.

2) It has no side effects. It is particularly suitable for those with impaired function of the heart, liver or kidney which renders drug anesthesia difficult and risky.

3) The patient is kept awake during the operation so the surgeon can check the patient's sensory and motor functions whenever necessary. This is particularly important in some neurological cases, for example, in operative intervention of acoustic neuroma, where injury of the facial nerves have been greatly reduced by application of "acupuncture anesthesia."

4) It increases the adaptive and regulatory ability of circulatory and immune functions. It is usually easier to keep the patient's blood pressure and pulse rate stable during the operation and achieve a faster rate of recovery.

III. Mechanism of Acupuncture Analgesia

Acupuncture analgesia is probably a more correct term than "acupuncture anesthesia." As a form of anesthesia, acupuncture raises the patient's pain threshold so an operation can be tolerated without distress. This is, in fact, a regulatory effect on physiological functions. Regulatory changes in the patient's body occur in response to needling stimulation at the site of acupoints. These changes alter the original functional state, increasing the pain threshold, minimizing pain response, and enhancing various vital functions such as circulation and immunity.

Studies on the mechanism at work in the elevation of the pain threshold have looked at activation of pain regulation and control system. Acupuncture interferes with the transmission of injurious stimuli from the operation site to the pain perception system. Various factors, including the nervous system and humoral regulation, are involved in this process. If acupuncture sensation is eliminated by injection of procaine at the acupoints site, no analgesic effect can be induced by acupuncture. In clinical practice, it is well recognized that the analgesic effect of acupuncture is closely related to acupuncture sensation. When, with acupuncture, there is a feeling of heaviness or distention, the injurious stimulation from the operation site will be restrained or inhibited. Recent studies have shown that inhibition of painful stimulation by non-painful stimulation occurs in the nervous system at various levels and involves the peripheral nerves, spinal cord, brain stem, thalamus and forebrain.

Apart from the nervous mechanism, other factors should be considered: The analgesic effect occurs after "an incubation period," not immediately after needling or having the acupuncture sensation; a long after-effect of analgesia is usually observed after cessation of acupuncture. In animal experiments, this analgesic effect can be abolished by injection of naloxone, a specific morphine antagonist; an analgesic effect has been reached in animals which receive no acupuncture but have cross perfusion of cerebrospinal fluid with other animals under acupuncture analgesia; and elevation of the level of a morphine-like substance has been found in the brain of animals under acupuncture analgesia. All these findings suggest a humoral mechanism — the release of morphine-like factor induced by acupuncture.

Acupuncture analgesia is a regulation of physiological functions. It can never lead to total loss of pain sensation or pain response. This limits the application of acupuncture analgesia and explains why some patients cannot tolerate surgery without another form of anesthesia. There are, however, many advantages to using acupuncture analgesia during surgery. Drug anesthesia can cause complete extirpation of pain, but there are side effects; acupuncture analgesia has no side effects, but extirpation of pain is incomplete. Combinations of acupuncture analgesia with the least amount of anesthetic drug, which bring anesthetic effect and avoid anesthetic accidents, have proven most satisfactory.

CHAPTER VIII
QI (VITAL ENERGY) AND *QIGONG*

Concept of *Qi*

The concept of *qi* is probably one of the most unique notions in traditional Chinese medicine, more so than even that of *yin-yang*. Like *yin-yang*, *qi* was derived from ancient Chinese philosophy, which considers it the most fundamental substance of the universe, to which everything is related. This naive understanding of natural phenomena was introduced into medicine, and the medical concept of *qi* came into being. Traditional Chinese medicine holds that *qi* is the fundamental substance of the human body; it explains various life processes with the movements and changes of *qi*. The complexity of this concept lies in its many implications. *Qi* in its physiological sense constitutes, replenishes and nourishes the human body. It particularly refers to the motive energy derived from the essential substance for various vital processes. Therefore, the word "*qi*" is often rendered into English as "vital energy." However, "*qi*" can also be used in a pathological sense, such as evil *qi*, which means the pathogenic factor. In this chapter, only essential *qi* in its physiological sense is discussed.

The concept of *qi* is even more complicated with respect to its actions. The main action of *qi* is to provide the force with which functional processes are carried on, including those physical, mental, and of the various visceral organs and tissues. In this context, *qi* is often classified according to what it acts on. For example, the heart-*qi* refers to the force with which the heart works and the blood circulates; the stomach-*qi* refers to the force with which the stomach functions. The heart-*qi* and stomach-*qi* can often be used as equivalents of the cardiac function and gastric function respectively. Besides this, *qi* has many other actions: It maintains normal functioning for resistance against disease. The *qi* possessing this action is called *zheng-qi* which means genuine energy or body resistance. The *qi* also warms the body and maintains normal

125

body temperature. The *qi* with this action is called *yang-qi*, which is approximate to the heat energy. The *qi* that protects the superficial portion of the body against the invasion of exogenous pathogens is called *wei-qi*, literally, the protecting force. The essential substance derived from food and drink to provide the body with nourishment is called *ying-qi* or nutrients. Metabolism of materials and energy also depends on the action of *qi*, including metabolism of blood, fluids and other essential materials. From the above, it can be understood why *qi* is so important in traditional Chinese medicine, and why the drugs to replenish *qi* must work in so many ways.

Qi is formed from the fresh air inhaled (i.e., oxygen), the nutrients from food, and the inborn primordial *qi* stored in the kidney (which implies genetic factors). *Qi* should circulate; the pathways along which it moves are the meridians and collaterals. Normal circulation of *qi* is one of the basic requirements of health. If there is stagnation of *qi* flow, a variety of morbid conditions may ensue. The circulation of *qi* is closely related with the mind. One of the common causes of *qi* stagnation is emotional upset. For example, anger may lead to dizziness, headache, distress in the hypochondriac regions, or distention in the stomach with impairment of appetite — all these ailments may be attributed to stagnation of *qi*. On the other hand, the mind can help *qi* circulate, of which the practice of *qigong* is most helpful.

General Methods of *Qigong*

Qigong is an exercise to regulate the mind and breathing in order to control or promote the flow of *qi*. Since *qi* plays such an important role in the vital processes of the human body, it is natural that regulation of *qi* flow can be used to preserve health and treat disease. *Qigong* practiced to prevent and treat disease is called medical *qigong*, which is different from physical exercise. The latter is aimed at building up health or restoring physical functioning by enhancing strength, while the former is focused on mobilization of functional potentialities by regulating the mind. In other words, physical exercise is purely somatic, while *qigong* therapy is generally psycho-somatic. Another important difference between physical exercise and *qigong* is that physical exercise expends energy by tensing the muscles and accelerating the heart beat and respiration, while *qigong* works to ease, still and regulate breathing to store up or accumulate energy in the body.

Medical *qigong* can be divided into two main categories: internal or endogenous *qigong* and external or exogenous *qigong*. The former is practiced by the patients themselves to preserve and promote their own health; the latter is performed by a *qigong* master to treat others' diseases. In this section, internal medical *qigong* is the main issue discussed.

Practicing internal *qigong* requires regulation of the mind, body and respiration, among which regulation of the mind is crucial. There are many kinds of internal *qigong*, some with motion and others without. In quiescent *qigong* (*qigong* without motion), adoption of a proper position is necessary. *Qigong* can be practiced while sitting still, standing upright, or lying on the back or side. The basic requirement is to stay comfortable and relaxed. *Qigong* with motion is usually the combination of *qigong* with physical exercise or self-massage.

There are also many ways to regulate respiration. In most cases, breathing should be natural, deep, slow, long, fine and even, with inhalation through the nose and exhalation through the mouth, but different patterns may be required for different purposes. For example, abdominal breathing and prolongation of inhalation is often helpful for promoting gastro-intestinal processes; prolongation of exhalation may help those with hypertension, pulmonary emphysema or glaucoma.

Whether with motion or without, the key point is regulation of the mind. Regulation of the mind means to remove all thoughts and focus on a certain region of the body, one of the points called *dantian* (literally, "elixir field"). There are three elixir fields: the lower one is located in the center of the abdomen about three inches below the umbilicus; the middle is located on the mid-line of the sternum between the nipples; and the upper is the region between the eyebrows. Each region has its own function, so, for example, concentration on the lower elixir field lowers blood pressure, while concentration on the upper raises it. Concentration on the lower elixir field is generally practiced, particularly for health care of the aged. As the body relaxes, the mind concentrates on the elixir field and all other thoughts are erased; respiration becomes deeper and gradually decreases in frequency. When the respiration rate is decreased to four or five times per minute, the subject falls into the so-called "*qigong* state."

The following are examples of internal *qigong*:

Pattern I (*Qigong* of Inner Cultivation)

1. *Preparation*:

(1) One should not be influenced or disturbed by the environment. The mind should be clear of thought.

(2) In any position, sitting or lying, the clothes should be loose so that respiration and blood circulation are free from restraint. The posture should be natural, without squaring the shoulders or pulling in the abdomen.

2. *Instructions*:

(1) Relaxation.

(a) Physical relaxation: Drink some water, empty the bowels and bladder, take off the hat, wrist-watch and glasses, loosen the clothes and belt, and relax the whole body, including the head, trunk and limbs.

(b) Mental relaxation: Begin with an easy mind.

(2) Posture. Select a comfortable and natural posture. The form selected is not important.

(a) Lying down. Lie on the side (either the right or the left) with the head slightly bent forward and placed comfortably on a pillow. If lying on the right side, extend the left arm naturally along the left (upper) side of the trunk with the left palm facing downward, placed on the left hip; bend the right arm at the elbow with the right palm facing upward and the fingers separated, placed on the pillow about six-seven cm from the head. Bend the waist a little bit, extend the right leg naturally with a slight bend at the knee; bend the left leg 120 degrees and rest it on the right leg.

(b) Sitting up. Sit upright on a bench with the legs apart at shoulder's width and knees bent at a 90-degree angle. Place the feet flat on the floor. (Adjust the height of the bench to meet these requirements.) The palms, facing upward, are placed at the middle third of the thighs, with the elbows naturally bent and relaxed.

(3) Silent recitation. "Recite" a short sentence in your mind. Start with a sentence of three words or a few syllables and gradually increase the number. Though there is no fixed pattern, those commonly used are: "I am still," "I am sitting (lying) still," "I am sitting (lying) very still," and so on.

Recitation should be coordinated with respiration. There are two methods: 1) Inhale with the first word, and exhale with the last; hold the breath in between; and 2) Recite the whole sentence in the pause between inhalation and exhalation. Either way, the more words in a sentence, the longer the pause in respiration.

(4) Breathing. Abdominal breathing is practiced. There are two methods: 1) Inhale and exhale through the nose. Lift the tongue to touch the palate while inhaling and lower it while exhaling. Inhalation should be natural without exertion, and the mind should be concentrated on the elixir field; and 2) Inhale through the mouth, using the mind to guide the air to the lower abdomen. Exhale naturally through the nose, followed by a pause for the sentence, during which time the tongue is touching the palate. After reciting the sentence, lower the tongue and inhale again.

(5) Concentration of the mind. The mind should be concentrated on the lower elixir field, free from all distractions. After repeated practice, a "tranquil" state will be reached.

Pattern II (Roborant *Qigong*)

1. *Preparation*: Same as those listed in Pattern I.
2. *Instructions*:
(1) Posture.

(a) Sitting cross-legged. Sit upright with the legs crossed. Do not square the shoulders. Place both hands in front of the lower abdomen with the four fingers of one hand on the palm of the other, one thumb on top of the other. If one is unable to sit cross-legged, the sitting form described in Pattern I may be adopted.

(b) Standing. Choose a peaceful environment where there is no noise and there is fresh air. Stand naturally and comfortably with the feet apart at shoulder's width and slightly bent, the head upright, the hands placed in front of the lower abdomen.

(2) Breathing. Breathe through the nose with the tip of the tongue lightly touching the palate. Use one of the following breathing patterns:

(a) Quiet breathing. Breathe naturally.

(b) Deep breathing. The breathing is deep, long, fine and even.

(c) Reverse breathing. Expand the chest and pull in the abdomen while inhaling, and pull in the chest and bulge the abdomen while exhaling.

(3) Concentrating the mind.

(a) During exhalation, guide the flow of *qi* downward from the perineum along the thighs, knees and shanks to the center of the soles.

(b) During inhalation, guide the flow of *qi* upward from the center of the soles along the shanks, knees and thighs to the perineum, until it reaches the lower elixir field, three inches below the umbilicus.

Physiological Changes During *Qigong*

1. The Brain

The human brain is an extremely complicated system, of which there are multiple states: normally, in waking, drowsy or sleeping state and abnormally, in hallucinatory or hypnotic state. The "*qigong* state" is different from those above. During *qigong* practice electroencephalograms show the following changes: after one or two minutes, the amplitude of alpha waves increases, first only in the occipital lobe, and then in the frontal lobe with decreased frequency. These changes are generally maintained throughout *qigong* practice. It has also been observed that the asymmetrical alpha waves between the two hemispheres become symmetrical. All these findings indicate that the "*qigong* state" is different from sleeping state, and *qigong* may improve physiological processes of the brain cells with improved synchronization. In fact, "*qigong* state" is not a state of inhibition but of oriented consciousness. This may explain why after practice one is usually in high spirits and able to think quickly and clearly; sight and hearing are also sharpened.

2. The Autonomic Nervous System

There may be physiological changes in the cardiovascular, respiratory and digestive systems during *qigong* practice. Since the functional processes of these systems are controlled by the autonomic nervous system, it is natural to suppose that *qigong* may effect this part of the nervous system. Tests of skin potential activity have been used to detect sympathetic results. Skin potential activities are synchronous and symmetrical on the right and left sides of healthy individuals, but asymmetry is typical in patients with mental or neurological diseases (such as schizophrenia, depression, hemiplegia, or brain trauma) and patients with lesions on one limb (such as injury to one arm or unilateral joint pain). In "*qigong* state," the skin potential activity becomes symmetrical, indicating better integration of the autonomic nervous system.

3. Respiration and Metabolism

During *qigong* practice, the respiration rate may be decreased to four or five times per minute. Under such circumstances, ventilation is decreased, but the subject does not feel suffocated. The explanation is that in *"qigong* state" oxygen consumption is much lower than even in sleeping state. The lowered metabolic rate and decreased energy consumption probably aid in the recovery of bodily functions.

4. The Cardiovascular System

In *"qigong* state" there are also functional changes in the cardiovascular system. *Qigong* often lowers blood pressure, particularly in those with hypertension, but elevates it in hypotensive patients. This regulatory effect is related to the form or pattern of *qigong*. For example, for lowering blood pressure, concentration must be focused on the lower part of the body (the lower elixir field or the center of the soles); sitting or standing may work better than lying down.

There may be changes in the heart rate during *qigong* practice — usually it lowers. In most cases, the blood vessels dilate, and the skin temperature of the middle finger rises by 2-3 ℃. Immediately after practice, the lower abdomen, waist and extremities may feel warm.

5. The Digestive System

In *"qigong* state" gastric peristalsis and evacuation are expedited, stomach tonus is increased and intestinal movements increase with intensified intestinal gurgling. Gastric and salivary secretion and activity of salivary amylase all increase.

6. The Blood and Immune System

Practicing *qigong* over a long time usually leads to increase of peripheral red blood cells, white blood cells and hemoglobin. Sometimes, these changes occur immediately after practice, probably due to massage of the liver and spleen by abdominal respiration. *Qigong* also promotes the phagocytosis of white blood cells and increases the lymphocyte transformation rate.

Treatment of Hypertension with *Qigong*

From the above, it can be seen that *qigong* may be utilized in the treatment of a wide spectrum of diseases. Hypertension in particular has been studied and the therapeutic effects of *qigong* repeatedly confirmed. A report from Shanghai Research Institute of Hypertension showed that a group of patients who practiced *qigong* aside from regular administration of hypotensors experienced better results than those of a comparable group treated with hypotensors alone. In the follow-up each year for four years thereafter, good therapeutic effect was found in 86.7-95.6% of those practicing *qigong* and in 70.7-76.6% of those receiving drug therapy alone. Similar results were obtained in six batches of clinical studies with 2,214 patients.

It has also been reported that *qigong* works well in the prognosis of hypertension. In a 20-year study of two comparable groups of hypertension patients, of the 104 patients who received regular drug therapy and practiced *qigong*, 16.3% suffered stroke and 11.5% died; but of the 100 patients who only received drug therapy, 30% suffered stroke and 23% died. In a series of 98 patients with essential hypertension complicated by coronary heart disease, a one-year follow-up showed that in 58.8% of those who practiced *qigong* electrocardiograms had improved, while such improvement only occurred in 21.6% of those who were treated with drug therapy alone. The above data indicates that *qigong* over time not only controls the blood pressure in patients with hypertension, but is also effective for treatment of coronary heart disease and prevention of stroke.

Studies have been done to determine the mechanisms at work:

1. Improvement of Cerebral Functions

Electroencephalography showed marked increase in amplitude and decrease in frequency of alpha waves in hypertension patients who practiced *qigong* while in "*qigong* state." No such changes were found in the patients who only received drug therapy when they were resting with their eyes shut.

2. Lowering of Sympathetic Hyperactivity

The level of norepinephrine, the sympathetic neurotransmitter, was estimated by assaying urinary excretion of its metabolites. Comparing patients who practiced *qigong* after practice and those who received only drug therapy after a rest of similar length, urinary excretion of metabolites of norepinephrine in the *qigong* group was much lower than the resting group. Since development of hypertension is closely associated with sympathetic hyperactivity and autonomic nervous imbalance, the regulatory action of *qigong* on the autonomic nervous functions undoubtedly plays an important role in the treatment of hypertension.

3. Improvement of Hemorheological Indices

Hemorheological changes such as increased blood viscosity and platelet aggregation with microcirculatory disorders are often encountered in hypertension patients. These are high risk factors for cardiovascular and cerebrovascular accidents, particularly myocardial infarction and cerebrovascular thrombosis. It has been reported that practice of *qigong* can reduce blood viscosity, restrain blood platelet aggregation, and improve micro-circulation, thus reducing the incidence of cerebrovascular accidents and mitigating coronary arterial complications in hypertension patients.

4. Regulation of Lipid and Carbohydrate Metabolism

Disorder of lipid metabolism with increased blood lipids is a major cause of atherosclerosis, and high blood sugar is a precipitating factor of cardiovascular disease. It has been reported that after *qigong* exercise, plasma triglyceride and total cholesterol levels were lowered, and the high-density-lipoprotein-cholesterol level raised. These changes help prevent atherosclerotic lesions of coronary and cerebral arteries. Blood sugar assayed before and after *qigong* exercise of hypertension patients who also suffered from diabetes mellitus showed marked reduction after practice. This suggests that *qigong* not only helps prevent cardiovascular disease, but may also work on diabetes mellitus. *Qigong* has been used by many diabetics with satisfactory results, especially by those with non-insulin-dependent diabetes mellitus.

Treatment of Other Diseases with *Qigong*

The indications of *qigong* are by no means confined to hypertension. Many other diseases, such as peptic ulcer, chronic gastritis, gastroptosis, bronchial asthma, neurosis and glaucoma have been effectively treated with this unique therapy. Although the clinical results have been confirmed, fewer studies have been done than on cases of hypertension.

Qigong Deviations

Qigong may produce abnormal psychosomatic responses, even mental disorder, if practiced inappropriately. These abnormal responses, or *qigong* deviations, generally fall into one of four groups:

1. Sensory Disturbance ("Adverse Flow of Qi")
This is the mildest form of *qigong* deviation, often manifested as a special sensation (the flow of *qi*) rushing to the head, distension at the elixir field, distress in the chest and feeling of suffocation. It is associated with nervousness, insomnia and disturbed sleep.

2. Motor Disturbance
In conjunction with sensory disturbance, the body may go out of control with tremor, odd movements of the limbs, and even strange behavior.

3. Mental Derangement
(1) "Overstate": In conjunction with sensory and motor disturbance, there may be mental disorder with incoherent speech, excitement, depression, fright or bewilderment.
(2) "State of being possessed": This may occur abruptly without sensory and motor disturbance. The common symptoms are hallucination, derangement of thought and delusion.

Qigong deviations are usually due to incorrect regulation of the mind to reach the "tranquil" state or control respiration. Proper coaching is a must to practice *qigong* safely.

About "Out-going Qi" ("External Qi")

In *qigong* practice, the flow of *qi* directed by the mind can be released from the body. This is a form of external *qigong*, and the *qi* sent out is called "out-going *qi*" or "external *qi*." The out-going *qi* can be used for various medical purposes, but in most cases, external *qi* is emitted not by the patient himself but from a healthy healer to the patient. One who can release directionally emitted external *qi* is called a "*qigong* master."

Qigong analgesia is probably one of the most conspicuous examples of this form of treatment. As with acupuncture, external *qi* can produce an analgesic effect when the *qi* is emitted to a patient who is suffering from pain. This effect is so remarkable that an experienced *qigong* master can alleviate even stubborn cancer pain. *Qigong* analgesia has also been tried as a kind of anesthesia in such surgical operations as removal of goiter.

During *qigong* analgesia, the master usually stands apart from the patient and emits external *qi* from the finger tips to a specific part of the patient's body. Since the fingers don't touch the patient and *qi* is invisible, it is easy to suspect the *qigong* master of using magic and the effect of the master's treatment merely the result of psychic or hypnotic influence. Recent research has clarified some of these suspicions.

Objective evidence of *qigong* analgesia has been obtained in animal experiments. It was demonstrated that the pain threshold of rats rose markedly when treated with external *qi*. Not only did the threshold rise during treatment, but it remained high for four hours thereafter.

As to the mechanisms involved, a clinical study revealed a distinct rise of the blood leucine enkephalin level during *qigong* analgesia. Leucine enkephalin is one of the smallest endorphins. Endorphins are endogenous morphine-like substances, widely present in the brain and nerves of the gastrointestinal tract. They are believed to play a major role in determining pain threshold. Marked increase of enkephalin suggests that this substance may mediate *qigong* analgesia.

A more complicated and interesting question is about the nature of external *qi*. This question is particularly challenging because it begs an explanation of *qi* in general. Though the theory of *qi* is a key point in traditional Chinese medicine, *qi* can hardly be studied but to look at the functional processes motivated by it in the human body. Some phenomena suggest the *qi* is in fact perceivable; for example, during acupuncture when the manipulator "hits" the *qi*, the subject may feel sore or numb, and the manipulator may feel tightening of the needle. These phenomena, however, are probably only detection of bodily response to *qi*, but not perception of *qi* itself. The case is entirely different with external *qi*. External *qi* emitted from the *qigong* master exists apart from the body before it reaches the recipient. It should therefore be able to be detected independently of other factors.

External *qi* has aroused interest not only among medical professionals, but also among biologists, chemists, physicists and those from other branches of the natural sciences. Extensive studies on the subject have been carried out in many academic institutions. Although there are still much debate, preliminary studies have provided clues to the existence of *qi*.

1) Infrared radiation has been detected in the external *qi* emitted by the *qigong* master. It has been demonstrated that a master can control the intensity of the infrared radiation from his own body as well as the intensity and distribution of infrared radiation on the receiver's body surface. Under the influence of external *qi*, the receiver may have a feeling of heat, heaviness, distention, numbness or itching in conjunction with the increase of infrared radiation. This infrared radiation from the *qigong* master is therefore different from that of non-living matter; it is thought to be a kind of informational flow that can activate and alter the infrared radiation of the receiver.

2) Superweak illumination is a biological phenomenon found in higher living beings. Intensified superweak illumination usually occurs before cell division. There is marked increase and decrease of superweak illumination in the *qigong* master's finger tips whence external *qi* is emitted: illumination increases markedly during emission of external *qi* and decreases immediately after conclusion of the practice.

Superweak illumination can also be used to detect internal *qi*. In a study of the meridians, transmission of internal *qi* was induced by needling and perceived by soreness, distention or numbness. The corresponding finger showed abrupt increase of illumination as soon as the internal *qi* had been touched.

3) Changes in laser-Raman spectrum have been observed with water, normal saline and glucose solution after irradiation by external *qi* emitted from a *qigong* master. When water was irradiated by external *qi*, an extra peak appeared in the spectrum and lasted for two hours. When glucose solution was irradiated by external *qi*, more complicated changes occurred, which indicated structural alteration of glucose molecules. The question now is whether or not these substances treated with external *qi* have different therapeutic effects from ordinary water, saline and glucose solution.

Research has shown that external *qi* is not imaginary. It seems to be a sort of energy consisting of infrared radiation, superweak illumination, microne flow, and magnetic and bioelectric waves which may cause various physical, chemical and biological reactions. The key is that this energy directed from the *qigong* master carries information from the master's mind by changes of the frequency. External *qi* is thus a sort of informational flow, and the effects produced by it are not simply due to the energy itself, but to the frequency changes of the energy flow controlled by the *qigong* master.

Biological effects of external *qi*, which may be more interesting to medical professionals, have also been demonstrated.

1. Effect of External *Qi* on Immune Functions

External *qi* has been shown to have a remarkable effect on immune functions: it increases the phagocytosis of macrophages in mice, and enhances primary immune response in rabbits by promoting antibody production and prolonging the period of this production. These findings suggest that external *qi* promotes both cellular and humoral immunity.

2. Anti-tumor Effect of External *Qi*

The effect of external *qi* on tumor cells has also been studied. External *qi* has been shown to destroy carcinoma cells in the human uterine cervix, adenocarcinoma cells in the human stomach, and ascites carcinoma cells in mice. The rate of extermination by one irradiation of external *qi* is about 35% for ascites carcinoma, 16-36% for carcinoma of uterine cervix, and 25% for carcinoma of stomach. The tumor cells affected by external *qi* went through processes of degeneration, swelling, nuclear solution and cellular necrosis.

With regard to the mechanisms of external *qi* in such cases, the following results are important: (1) External *qi* enhances the levels of serum interleukin-2, interferon and lymphotoxin. (2) External *qi* enhances the level of plasma cAMP. As all work to control cancer this may help explain why *qigong*, both internal and external, can prolong a cancer patient's life.

3. Anti-bacterial Effect of External *Qi*

Remarkable bacteriocidal or bacteriostatic effects of external *qi* have been demonstrated on B. coli, Streptococcus, Bacillus dysenteriae and Bacillus pyocyaneus. Most interesting is the different results produced by different kinds of external *qi*. An experienced *qigong* master not only can inhibit the growth of bacteria, but can also promote their growth by altering the emission of external *qi*.

These findings may seem inconceivable, as they can hardly be explained by contemporary natural science, but the experiments were carried out in such famous academic institutions as Qinghua University, China Academy of Traditional Chinese Medicine, Chinese Academy of Medical Sciences, Beijing College of Traditional Chinese Medicine, Chinese Institute of Aerospace Medicine, and Shanghai Qigong Institute. Although many questions remain, the preliminary data suggest a greater potential in human beings than what has been recognized by contemporary physiology.

CHAPTER IX
DIETOTHERAPY IN TRADITIONAL CHINESE MEDICINE

Diet is of great significance in the preservation of health and treatment of disease. Chinese dietotherapy is founded on the basis of traditional medicine and includes medicinal materials as food. Traditional dietotherapy is thus not confined to the food recommended or prohibited in a certain disease. Most noteworthy is the so-called medicinal diet, which is composed of medicinal materials and food thought to have a therapeutic effect. Prepared according to recipes based on traditional medical theories, a medicinal diet is both delicious food and therapeutic medicine.

The medicinal diet can be traced to ancient times. There is a saying in traditional Chinese medicine: "Medicine and food are of the same origin," as much of both originate from plants. In fact, it is difficult to draw a line between medicinal materials and food. Many flowers, fruits, seeds, leaves, stems and roots can be used as both. This includes flavorings and seasonings, such as dates, honey, hawthorn fruit, black plum, longan aril, walnut, phaseolus seed, Job's-tears seed, lotus seed, euryale seed, ginger, cinnamon, safflower, pagodatree flower, capsella, poria and platycodon root. In *Ben Cao Gang Mu* (*Compendium of Materia Medica*) many foodstuffs are included.

Taste or flavor is both a criterion to describe the quality of food, and also a means of medicinal classification. Generally speaking, medicines can be classified into five or six categories according to the taste, i.e., pungent, sweet, sour, bitter, and salty; there are also medicines with mild taste or no taste. As medicines of different tastes usually have different actions, and those of the same taste may have similar actions, in Chinese materia medica, taste is a criterion for classification of pharmacological actions. The following describes general actions of medicines of different tastes:

The Five Tastes
— Pungent, Sweet, Sour, Bitter and Salty

Medicines of pungent flavor usually disperse (as diaphoresis) and promote flow of *qi* and blood. For example, Rhizoma Zingiberis Recens (fresh ginger) is used to induce diaphoresis in colds, Herba Menthae (peppermint) to relieve upper respiratory infection, Pericarpium Citri Reticulatae Viride (tangerine peel) and Fructus Amomi (amomum fruit) to promote *qi* of the *spleen* and stomach (i.e., promote digestion), and Radix Angelicae Sinensis (Chinese angelica root) and Rhizoma Ligustici Chuanxiong (chuanxiong rhizome) to promote blood flow and remove blood stasis.

Medicines of sweet taste usually tonify and relieve colic. For example, Radix Ginseng (ginseng) and Radix Astragali (astragalus root) replenish vital energy; Radix Ophiopogonis (ophiopogon root), Fructus Lycii (wolfberry fruit) and Carapax Trionycis (turtle shell) replenish essential substances; Radix Glycyrrhizae (licorice), Saccharum Granorum (malt extract) and Fructus Ziziphi Jujubae (Chinese date) relieve colic pain in the gastrointestinal tract.

Medicines of sour taste usually act as an astringent. For example, Fructus Chebulae (chebula fruit) and Fructus Mume (black plum) are effective for treating chronic diarrhea, Fructus Schisandrae (schisandra fruit) and Fructus Rosae Laevigatae (fruit of cherokee rose) for treating excessive sweating.

Medicines of bitter taste usually remove dampness and catharsis. For example, Rhizoma Coptidis (coptis root) and Radix Gentianae (Chinese gentian) eliminate heat and damp (inflammation and exudation); and Rhizoma et Radix Rhei (rhubarb) removes heat and damp through catharsis.

Medicines of salty taste usually soften hard masses and induce laxation. For example, Sargassum (seaweed) and Thallus Laminariae seu Eckloniae (laminaria) are used to treat goiter and scrofula; mirabilite (sodium sulfate) is used as a laxative.

The principle of classifying medicines according to taste is derived from the study of food with different tastes. Quite a few of the medicinal materials listed above are also used as food. In fact, food of a certain taste usually has similar actions as those listed above. Food can thus be used to restore balance, or if taken to excess, it may produce an adverse effect. Too much sour food, for example, may cause astringency, and too much spicy food may cause dispersion. It is better to avoid too much of one taste. An important principle in Chinese cuisine is the modulation of tastes in, for example, such dishes as hot and sour soup, sweet and sour fish. The proper combination of flavors not only makes the food more delicious, but also neutralizes possible adverse effects.

The Four Properties
— Hot, Warm, Cool and Cold

In *Materia Medica*, the basic properties of medicines are generally classified into four or five groups: hot, warm, cool, cold, and neutral (neither warm nor cool). Among these, hot and warm are only different by degree, and so are cool and cold. Generally speaking, there are therefore two main categories of medicines: those hot in nature and those cold in nature. This classification is related to the general classification of syndromes, which divides all into either cold syndromes or heat syndromes, though some are of both cold and heat, and some exhibit properties of neither.

Cold syndrome is characterized by pallor with aversion to cold, cold limbs, loose stools, white tongue coating and slow pulse. If there is pain, it is aggravated by cold and alleviated by warmth; if there is expectoration, the sputum is whitish and thin; saliva secretion is either sufficient or in excess. The patient feels no thirst and prefers hot drinks. Heat syndrome is characterized by a flushed face with general fever or feverishness, aversion to heat, thirst with scanty secretion of saliva, constipation, parched lips, reddened tongue with yellowish coating, and rapid pulse. If there is pain, it is aggravated by heat and alleviated by cold; if there is expectoration, the sputum is thick, yellowish or purulent.

Medicines indicated in the treatment of cold syndromes are believed to be hot or warm in property, and those indicated in the treatment of heat syndrome to be cold or cool in property. This principle is of crucial importance in traditional therapeutics because the wrong medicine may aggravate the disease or cause an adverse response.

Food can also be classified in the same manner.

1. Food hot or warm in property:
(1) Meat: beef, chicken, mutton, shrimp, snake.

(2) Vegetables: carrot, onion, garlic, chives, rape, coriander, fragrant-flowered garlic.
(3) Fruits: apricot, orange.
(4) Others: brown sugar, flour, ewe milk, pepper, ginger.

2. Food cool or cold in property:
(1) Meat: pork, oyster, duck, goose, rabbit.
(2) Vegetables: celery, spinach, cucumber, balsam pear, eggplant, tomato, white gourd, mung bean sprouts, bamboo shouts.
(3) Fruits: pear, water melon, pomelo, persimmon, banana.
(4) Others: mung bean, peppermint.

3. Food mild in property:
(1) Meat: carp, cuttlefish.
(2) Vegetables: carrot.
(3) Fruits: grape, peach, plum, apple.
(4) Others: rice (round-grained nonglutinous), flour, corn, broomcorn millet, soybean, red bean.

How were these properties determined? Primarily through experience in daily life and treatment of disease. Food is believed to be hot or warm if it makes one feel comfortable or gives relief in the cold season or in the course of a disease with cold syndrome. That which makes one feel comfortable or gives relief in the hot season or in the course of a disease with heat syndrome is believed to be cold or cool in property. As with medicines, food of the wrong property, particularly if taken for a long time or in large quantity, may cause an adverse response. For example, spicy hot food may cause constipation or epistaxis when eaten in a dry hot season; it is usually not tolerated by patients with acute fever. Too much celery, cucumber or balsam pear eaten in a cold season or by a patient with cold syndrome may result in loose stools with abdominal pain or aggravation of the syndrome.

Food is also believed to have therapeutic effects. It can cause diaphoresis, eliminate heat, dispel cold, induce laxation, replenish essential substances, reinforce vital functions, regulate the flow of qi and promote digestion. It can, in other words, be used as medicine.

Diet to Combat Pathogenic Factors*

From the perspective of traditional Chinese medicine, disease is a process of confrontation between the body and pathogenic factors. Treatment can be generally classified into two categories: those to eliminate pathogenic factors and those to strengthen body resistance. The former includes diaphoresis, laxation or catharsis, antipyresis, antibiosis, detoxication, diuresis, etc. The latter refers primarily to the actions of tonics. The following are examples of the first category.

1. Diaphoretic Tea

Diaphoretic tea is suitable for patients with colds or upper respiratory infection in the early stages. Generally speaking, colds and upper respiratory infection are of two types:

(1) Cold type: Immediately after catching a cold, there is chilliness, headache and pain. The most common recipe for relief at this stage is "ginger tea," a combination of 5-10g of sliced fresh ginger and brown sugar boiled in water for two-three minutes, which is taken warm.

(2) Heat type: This usually occurs in the early stage of upper respiratory infection and is manifested by chills and fever, sore throat, and reddened tongue with yellowish coating. Mulberry, chrysanthemum and lophatherum tea is recommended. Mulberry leaf (Folium Mori) 5g, chrysanthemum flower (Flos Chrysanthemi) 5g, peppermint (Herba Menthae) 3g, lophatherum (Herba Lophatheri) 30g, cogongrass rhizome (Rhizoma Imperatae) 30g and sugar 20g are boiled in water for two minutes. The drink is taken cool.

2. Laxative Candy

Laxative candy is taken for relief of constipation due to consumption of intestinal fluid, particularly in the aged. Mulberry (Fructus Mori) is often used for this purpose. It can be made into candy according to the following recipe: Sugar 50g and powdered dried mulberry 200g are heated until the sugar melts and formed into about 100 pieces

---

* The herbs used in a medicinal diet are described with the English name first and the Latin name in paratheses, for many are available in grocery stores.

of candy. Mulberry made into paste with honey is even more effective than the candy.

3. *Digestive Extract*

An extract for promoting digestion and removing retained gastric content can be made according to the following recipe: Charred medicated leaven (Massa Fermentata Medicinalis), charred crataegus fruit (Fructus Crataegi) and charred germinated barley (Fructus Hordei Germinatus), 10g of each, and sugar 30g are stewed in water for 15 minutes and then filtered. This extract is good for relieving indigestion with belching, sour eructation and epigastric distention.

4. *Carminative Areca*

Carminative areca is prepared according to the following recipe: Areca nut (Semen Arecae) 200g, tangerine peel (Pericarpium Citri Reticulatae) 20g, cloves (Flos Caryophylli), round cardamon seed (Semen Cardamomi) and amomum fruit (Fructus Amomi), 10g of each, are simmered in water with a bit of salt until dried. The areca is then cut into pieces as large as soybeans. Chewing carminative areca after each meal stimulates digestion, arrests sour eructation and relieves epigastric distention.

5. *Candied Kernel*

The recipe for preparing candied kernels is as follows: Simmer stir-fried apricot kernel 250g in water for one hour, add walnut kernel 250g and continue to simmer until dried, then add honey 500g and mix thoroughly. Candied kernel relieves chronic cough and asthma.

6. *Diuretic Porridge*

This porridge is made of Job's-tears seed (Semen Coicis) 50g and rice 150g simmered in water. It has a diuretic action and can be used to treat edema.

7. *Antipyretic Juice*

Pulp of watermelon 1,500g with the seeds removed and tomato 1,000g are mixed into a juice for patients with fever and thirstiness.

Diet for Strengthening Body Resistance

Diet for improving the constitution and strengthening body resistance is the main thrust of Chinese dietotherapy. "Tonic food" can be divided into similar groups as tonic drugs: *yin*-replenishing, *yang*-invigorating, *qi*-replenishing, and blood-replenishing. A tonic diet is used widely to treat chronic disease and preserve good health.

1. *Yin*-replenishing Medicinal Diet

This kind of diet is usually recommended to those with *yin* deficiency manifested by emaciation, dizziness, irritability, dryness in the mouth and throat, and insomnia. The medicinal herbs commonly used in the *yin*-replenishing diet are: fragrant solomonseal rhizome (Rhizoma Polygonati Odorati), ophiopogon root (Radix Ophiopogonis), asparagus root (Radix Asparagi), glehnia root (Radix Glehniae), lily bulb (Bulbus Lilii), wolfberry fruit (Fructus Lycii), and mulberry (Fructus Mori). They can be added to cooked food, as shown in the following examples:

(1) *Stewed pork with glehnia*

Stew glehnia root (Radix Glehniae), fragrant solomonseal rhizome (Rhizoma Polygonati Odorati), Chinese yam (Rhizoma Dioscoriae) and lily bulb (Bulbus Lilii), 15g of each, and lean pork 500g in water. Add the desired amount of salt or sauce, and eat everything. Stewed pork with glehnia is effective for treating *yin* deficiency with weakness, thirstiness and excessive sweating.

(2) *Lily soup with egg-yolk*

Soak 45g of lily bulb (Bulbus Lilii) in water overnight. Throw out the water, and boil lily bulbs until soft enough to eat. Add one egg yolk and sugar or other flavorings to the soup. Daily consumption will relieve nervousness and irritability.

(3) *Wolfberry gruel*

Boil wolfberry fruit (Fructus Lycii) 25g and rice 60g in water to make a gruel. Daily consumption is good for the aged with weak constitution and for those in convalescence after a severe illness.

2. *Yang*-invigorating Medicinal Diet

This kind of diet is recommended to those with *yang* deficiency manifested by general weakness accompanied with aversion to cold, cold limbs, loose stools or impotence. The medicinal herbs commonly used in preparing a *yang*-invigorating diet are: Curculigo rhizome (Rhizoma Curculiginis), epimedium (Herba Epimedii), cynomorium (Herba Cynomorii), morinda root (Radix Morindae Officinalis), eucommia bark (Cortex Eucommiae), and cordyceps (Cordyceps). They can be added to cooked food as illustrated by the following examples:

(1) *Cynomorium porridge*

Rinse cynomorium (Herba Cynomorii) 15g and cut it into thin slices. Boil it with rice 30g in water to make porridge. Daily consumption is effective for impotence, seminal emission, constipation, and aching of the lower back, particularly in the aged.

(2) *Epimedium wine*

Immerse epimedium (Herba Epimedii) 30g in 500 ml of wine for seven days. Drink 20-30 ml of the wine two-three times a day. It is good for impotence and aching of the back and knees with aversion to cold.

(3) *Cistanche and mutton soup*

Rinse cistanche (Herba Cistanchis) 15g in water and then in wine to remove the dark juice. Cut it into thin slices and boil it with mutton in water to make a soup. Add salt and other flavorings. Daily consumption is good for impotence, seminal emission, lower back pain and frequent urination.

3. *Qi*-replenishing Medicinal Diet

This kind of diet is recommended to those with *qi* deficiency manifested by general weakness accompanied with lassitude, shortness of breath, loss of appetite, and spontaneous sweating. The medicinal herbs commonly used in preparing a *qi*-replenishing diet are ginseng, astragalus root, pilose asiabell root, Chinese yam, white atractylodes rhizome and jujube (Chinese date). They can be added to cooked food as illustrated by the following examples:

(1) *Astragalus and pork soup*

Boil astragalus root 30g, ten Chinese dates, lean pork, salt and other flavorings in water. This soup is good for general weakness with spontaneous sweating.

(2) *Ginseng soup*

Cut 1-2g of American ginseng into thin slices and add them to vegetable soup for replenishing vital energy.

(3) *Astragalus porridge*

Boil astragalus root (Radix Astragali) 30g, wrapped in a piece of gauze, and polished glutinous rice 30g in water to make porridge. Remove the astragalus root before serving. Daily consumption will help prevent colds and treat albuminuria in patients with nephritis.

4. Blood-replenishing Medicinal Diet

This kind of diet is recommended to those with blood deficiency manifested by pallor, dizziness, palpitation, amenorrhea or insomnia. The medicinal herbs commonly used in preparing a blood-replenishing diet are: Chinese angelica root (Radix Angelicae Sinensis), white peony root (Radix Paeoniae Alba), longan aril (Arillus Longan) and prepared rehmannia root (Radix Rehmanniae Praeparata). They can be added to cooked food as illustrated in the following examples:

(1) *Chinese angelica and mutton soup*

Cut 500g of mutton into small pieces. Stew it with Chinese angelica root (Radix Angelicae Sinensis), astragalus root (Radix Astragali) and pilose asiabell root (Radix Codonopsis Pilosulae), 25g of each, wrapped in a piece of gauze, to make a thick soup. When the mutton becomes tender, add 25g of fresh ginger slices and salt; cook until the mutton melts in the mouth. This soup is effective for treating weakness with anemia, particularly for postpartum anemia.

(2) *Longan and lotus seed gruel*

Boil longan aril 15g, lotus seed 10g and rice 100g in water to make a gruel. Daily consumption is an effective treatment for anemia.

(3) *Steamed chicken with astragalus root*

One chicken; astragalus root (Radix Astragali) 30g, salt 1.5g, rice wine 15g, green onion and fresh ginger, 10g of each, broth 500g and pepper powder 2g. Boil astragalus root for a few minutes and rinse it with cold water. Cut the root into segments about 6 cm long, and split each segment lengthwise into two. Place the root into the chicken's abdominal cavity, and steam the chicken with salt, rice wine, green onion, ginger and broth for 1.5-2 hours. Add pepper before serving.

5. Medicinal Diet for Replenishing both *Qi* and Blood

(1) *Astragalus and date soup*

Boil astragalus root (Radix Astragali) 30g and dates 30g in water to make a soup. Eat the soup and dates but not the root. Daily consumption will promote recovery after disease with deficiency of both *qi* and blood.

(2) *Stewed meat with Chinese angelica root and pilose asiabell root*

Stew meat (pork or beef) with pilose asiabell root (Radix Codonopsis Pilosulae) 30g, Chinese angelica root (Radix Angelicae Sinensis) and ten dates. Consumption of the meat, dates and soup is effective for restoration of health from deficiency of *qi* and blood.

All the recipes listed above will have a certain effect if used properly. In China, there are restaurants where medicinal dishes are served. The recipes used are not mentioned here for they require specialized techniques beyond the scope of this book.

Food Taboos

The earliest records of food taboos can be found in *Canon of Medicine*, as the chapter "The Five Flavors" states: "Spicy food is prohibited with *liver* disease; salty food is prohibited with *heart* disease; sour food is prohibited with *spleen* disease;..." In *Jin Kui Yao Lue* (*Synopsis of Prescriptions of the Golden Chamber*), written at the beginning of the 3rd century by Zhang Zhongjing, one of the most influential physicians in the history of Chinese medicine, food taboos are described in more detail. He calls for abstention from salt during edema, and abstention from greasy food if there is jaundice or diarrhea.

As mentioned above, food, like medicine, is categorized according to hot, warm, cool and cold properties. The rule in dietotherapy is that food hot or warm in property is beneficial for treating cold syndromes and food cool or cold in property beneficial for heat syndromes. Likewise, food cold in property should be avoided with cold syndromes (for example, cucumber and banana may aggravate chronic diarrhea) and that hot in property should be avoided with hot syndromes (garlic and chilli may aggravate constipation).

There are also taboos for specific diseases. For example, patients with bronchial asthma are usually advised to abstain from seafood such as shrimp, crab and fish; patients with cough and profuse expectoration are advised to avoid greasy food; patients with senile cataract are advised to abstain from garlic and chives.

The quantity of food eaten is also an important factor. Food warm or cool in property is milder than that which is hot or cold, but a large quantity may also cause harmful effects.

Another point worth mentioning is the temperature of food.

Food hot or cold in property does not indicate temperature. However, there is some relationship in this regard. The cold property of food is enhanced if it is eaten cold, and the hot property enhanced if it is eaten hot.

INDEX

Abnormal fetal position, auriculo-acupressure correction of 113
ABO hemolysis 38-40
　herbal treatment of 39-40
　prevention of 39-40
Acanthopanax root 35, 64, 68
Aconite root 35
Acupuncture analgesia 121-124
　advantages of 122
　disadvantages of 122
　mechanism of 123
Acupuncture and moxibustion 106-124
　contraindications of 116
　indications of 110-116
　methods of 108-110
　technique of 108-110
　therapeutic mechanism of 117-121
　　functional state of the patient 117
　　intensity of stimulation 118
　　selection of acupoints 119
Acupuncture points 106
Acupuncture treatment 111-123
　bronchial asthma 116
　cerebral infarction 111-112
　leukopenia, chemotherapy-induced 114
　male infertility 114
　obesity 115
　pain 121-122
Acute infections 43-59
　differentiation of syndromes in 43-45
　herbal treatment of 45-47
"Adaptogen-like" substances 36
Allergic rhinitis 37-38
　herbal treatment of 37-38
Anemarrhena rhizome 44, 48
Artemisine 59
Ass-hide gelatin 65, 66
Astragalus root 29, 30, 34, 64, 66, 89
Auriculo-acupressure correction of abnormal fetal position 113

Ben Cao Gang Mu (*Compendium of Materia Medica*) 4
Ben Cao Jing Ji Zhu (*Commentaries on Materia Medica*) 3
Bian Que 1
Blood 15
　stasis 6, 20
Body fluid 15
Bronchial asthma, acupuncture treatment of 116
Bupleurum root 44, 48

Calculus bovis (ox gallstone) 44, 48
Cancer 93-105
　blood-stasis-removing therapy of 97
　body-resistance-strengthening therapy of 96-97

151

herbal medication of   95-105
herbal medication with chemotherapy of   99-103
herbal medication with radiotherapy of   99-103
toxic-heat-clearing therapy of   97-98
traditional concept of   93-95
Canon of Medicine   1
Cerebral infarction, acupuncture treatment of   111
Chemotherapy-induced leukopenia, acupuncture treatment of   114
Chinese angelica root   33, 64, 68
Chinese date   35
Chinese traditional gerontology   82-92
Chronic bronchitis   71-73
  etiology and pathogenesis of   72
  herbal treatment of   72
Chronic gastritis   73-75
  traditional treatment of   74-75
Chrysanthemum   44, 48
Classic on the Pulse   2
Colla corii asini (ass-hide gelatin)   65, 66
Cold   19
  endogenous   19
  exogenous   19
Commentaries on Materia Medica   3
Compendium of Materia Medica   4
Coptis root   34, 36, 46, 51, 52
Cornu cervi pantotrichum (pilose deerhorn)   66, 70
  rhinoceri (rhinoceros horn)   45, 49
Cortex phellodendri (phellodendron bark)   36, 46

Dampness   19
  endogenous   19
  exogenous   19
Dandelion herb   46, 51, 52
Dang Gui Long Hui Wan (Pill of Chinese Angelica, Gentian and Aloe)   98
Dantian (elixir field)   127
Decoction for Clearing Heat from the *Ying* System   47
Decoction of Four Noble Ingredients   103
Deerhorn, pilose   66, 70
Deficiency syndrome   21-22, 61-62
  deficiency of blood   22
  deficiency of *qi*   21
  deficiency of *yang*   22
  deficiency of *yin*   22
Depression, electro-acupuncture treatment of   112
Diabetes mellitus   76-78
  dietotherapy of   77
  etiology and pathogenesis of   77
  herbal treatment of   77-78
Dietotherapy   139-148
Diphenyldiester   57
Dodder seed   30, 35, 80
Dryness   19
Dyer's woad root   46

Ephedra   32
Epimedium   66, 68
Electro-acupuncture treatment of

152

depression 112
Elixir field 127
Essence 15
  congenital 15
  reproductive 15
  vital (see *Qi*)
Exterior syndrome 43

Fire 19
  endogenous 20
  exogenous 19
Five elements 11-12
  doctrine of 11-12
Five tastes 140-141
  of food 140
  of medicines 140
Fleeceflower root 35, 68
Flos chrysanthemi (chrysanthemum) 44, 48
  lonicerae (honeysuckle flower) 33, 51
Folium mori (mulberry leaf) 48
  perillae (perilla leaf) 33
Food taboos 148
Forsythia fruit 33, 51
Four properties 141-142
  of food 141
  of medicines 141
Fructus forsythiae (forsythia fruit) 33, 51
  ligustri lucidi (lucid ligustrum fruit) 65
  lycii (wolfberry fruit) 34, 65, 66, 80
  psoraleae (psoralea fruit) 66, 68
  schisandrae (schisandra fruit) 34, 57
  ziziphi jujubae (Chinese date) 35

Ganoderma lucidum (lucid ganoderma) 30, 34, 66
Gerontology, Chinese traditional 82-92
Ginseng 30, 31, 35, 63, 66, 68, 89
Green chiretta 46, 52
Guben Wan (Pill for Strengthening Constitution) 73
Gypsum 44, 48
Gypsum fibrosum 44, 48

Half-exterior half-interior syndrome 44
Hay fever (see Allergic rhinitis)
Heart 13
Herba
  androgarphitis (green chiretta) 46, 52
  artemisiae chinghao (sweet wormwood) 59
  artemisiae scopariae (oriental wormwood) 56
  ephedrae (ephedra) 32
  epimedii (epimedium) 66, 69
  houttuyniae (houttuynia) 46, 52
  oldenlandiae (oldenlandia) 33
  taraxaci (dandelion herb) 46, 51, 52
  schizonepetae (schizonepeta) 43, 48
  violae (viola herb) 46, 49, 51
Herbal immunomodulators 34-37
  immunopotentiator 29-32
  immunosuppressor 32-34
Herbs

153

blood-activating 23
heat-clearing and detoxifying 29
immunomodulating 34-36
immunopotentiating 29-32
immunosuppressing 32-34
wind-dispelling 18
with antibacterial effect 48, 49
with antipyretic effect 48
with antiviral effect 48
with diaphoretic effect 48
Honeysuckle flower 33, 50
Houttuynia 46
Huang Di Nei Jing (*The Yellow Emperor's Canon of Medicine*) 1
Hypertension, *qigong* treatment of 131-133
Hyperthyroidism 78-80
herbal treatment of 79-80
pathogenesis of 79

Indirubin 98
Influenza 54-55
herbal treatment of 54-55
Interior syndrome 44-45

Jade-screen Powder 30-31
Jiang Tang Jia Pian (Tablet for Reducing Blood Sugar No. A) 77
Jin Kui Yao Lue Fang Lun (*Synopsis of Prescriptions of the Golden Chamber*) 2

Kidney 4, 13

Ledebouriella root 43
Leukopenia, chemotherapy-induced, acupuncture treatment of 114
Liquorice 35
Liuwei Dihuang Wan (Pill of Six Ingredients with Rehmannia) 104-105
Liver 13
Lucid ganoderma 30, 34, 66
Lucid ligustrum fruit 65
Lung 13

Mai Jing (Classic on the Pulse) 2
Malaria 58-59
Male infertility 80-81
acupuncture treatment of 114
herbal treatment of 80-81
Medicinal diet 139
antipyretic 144
blood-replenishing 147
diaphoretic 143
diuretic 144
qi-replenishing 146
yang-invigorating 145
yin-replenishing 145
laxative 143
Meridians 106
twelve regular 106
extra 107
fourteen 107
yang 10
yin 10
Mulberry leaf 48

Nei Jing (see *Huang Di Nei Jing*)

Obesity, acupuncture treatment of 115
Oldenlandia 33
Ophiopogon root 65

Oriental wormwood 56
Ox gallstone 44, 48

Pain, acupuncture treatment of 121-122
Pathogenic factors 17
   endogenous 17
   exogenous 17
Phellodendron bark 36, 46
Perilla leaf 33
Phlegm 20-21
   invisible 21
   visible 21
Pill for Replenishing Kidney Qi 76
Pill of Chinese Angelica, Gentian and Aloe 98
Pill of Five Kinds of Seeds for Bringing Forth Offspring 80, 90
Pill of Six Ingredients with Rehmannia 104-105
Polise asiabell root 31, 34, 66, 68
Pilose deerhorn 66, 70
Polyporus umbellatus polysaccaride 57
Powder of Lonicera and Forsythia 46, 54
Psoralea fruit 66, 69
Pulsatilla root 46

Qi (vital energy) 14, 125-126
   acquired 14
   concept of 125
   deficiency of 21-22
   external 134-138
   formation of 126
   inborn 14
   physiological 14
   stagnation of 20
   wei-qi (protecting energy) 126
   yang-qi (heat energy) 126
   zheng-qi (genuine energy) 125
Qigong 126-138
   external 127
   general methods of 126-127
   inner cultivating 87, 128
   internal 127
   quiescent 127
   roborant 87, 129
Qigong state 127, 130-131
   autonomic nervous system in 130
   blood system in 131
   brain in 130
   cardiovascular system in 131
   digestive system in 131
   immune system in 131
   metabolism in 131
   physiological changes in 130-131
   respiration in 131
Qigong treatment 131-133
   hypertension 131-133
Qing Ying Tang (Decoction for Clearing Heat from the Ying System) 47
Qinghaosu (Artemisine) 59

Radix acanthopanacis senticosi (acanthopanax root) 35, 64, 68
   aconiti (aconite root) 34
   angelicae sinensis (Chinese angelica root) 33, 64, 68
   astragali (astragalus root) 29, 30, 34, 64, 66, 89
   bupleuri (bupleurum root) 44,

155

codonopsis pilosulae (pilose asiabell root) 31, 34, 66, 68
coptidis (coptis root) 34, 36, 51, 52
ginseng 30, 31, 35, 63, 66, 68, 89
glycyrrhizae (liquorice) 35
isatidis (dyer's woad root) 46
ledebouriellae (ledebouriella root) 43
ophiopogonis (ophiopogon root) 65
polygoni multiflori (fleeceflower root) 35, 68
pulsatillae (pulsatilla root) 46
rehmanniae (rehmannia root) 35, 66
rehmanniae praeparata (prepared rehmannia root) 64
salviae miltiorrhizae (red sage root) 33, 97
scutellariae (scutellaria root) 34, 44, 46, 51, 52
Radix et rhizoma rhei (rhubarb) 36, 48, 52-53, 56
Red sage root 33, 97
Rehmannia root 35, 66
  prepared 64
Revised Materia Medica 3
Rhinoceros horn 45, 49
Rhizoma anemarrhenae (anemarrhena rhizome) 44, 48
  atractylodis macrocephalae (white atractylodes rhizome) 66, 70
  coptidis (coptis root) 34, 36, 51, 52
  polygonati (Siberian solomonseal rhizome) 89
Rhubarb 36, 48, 52-53, 56

Schisandra fruit 34, 57
Schizonepeta 43, 48
Scleroderma (see Systemic sclerosis)
Scutellaria root 34, 44, 52
Semen cuscutae (dodder seed) 30, 35, 80
Senility 83-92
  cause of 83
  prevention of 84-92
    adaptation to nature 84
    health-preserving exercises 87
    herbal medication 88
    maintenance of calm and cheerful mood 84
    preservation of vital essence 86
    rational diet 85
Shang Han Lun (*Treatise on Febrile Diseases*) 2
Shen Nong Ben Cao Jing (*Shen Nong's Herbal*) 2
Shen Qi Wan (Pill for Replenishing Kidney Qi) 76
Si Junzi Tang (Decoction of Four Noble Ingredients) 102
Siberian solomonseal rhizome 89
Solution of Five Kinds of Seeds for Bringing Forth Offspring 90
Spleen 13
Stagnation of qi 20
Sun Simiao 85
Sweet wormwood 59
Syndrome
  cold 5
  deficiency 21-22, 61-62

differentiation in acute infections 43-45
excess 22-23
exterior 43-44
half-exterior half-interior 44
heat 5
interior 44
Synopsis of Prescriptions of the Golden Chamber 2
Systemic sclerosis 40-41
   herbal treatment of 41

Tablet for Reducing Blood Sugar No. A 77
Tablet for Relieving *Xiaoke* 78
Tonics 61-81
   actions of 66-70
      on adaptability 67
      on endocrine system 68
      on immune functions 66-67
      on metabolism 68
      roborant 69
   blood tonics 64-65
   indications of 69
   qi tonics 29, 63-64
   yang tonics 65-66
   yin tonics 29, 65
Treatise on Febrile Diseases 2

Viola herb 46, 49, 50
Viral hepatitis 55-58
   herbal treatment of 56-58
Vital energy (see *Qi*)
Vital essence 15

White atractylodes rhizome 66, 69
Wholism 11-12
Wind 17

endogenous 17
exogenous 17
Wolfberry fruit 34, 65, 66, 80
Wu Zi Yan Zong Wan (Pill of Five Kinds of Seeds for Bringing Forth Offspring) 80, 90
Wu Zi Yan Zong Ye (Solution of Five Kinds of Seeds for Bringing Forth Offspring) 90

Xiaoke 76
Xiao Ke Ping Pian (Tablet for Relieving *Xiaoke*) 78
Xin Xiu Ben Cao (Revised Materia Medica) 3

Yang 5, 9-10
   exuberance of 5
   insufficiency (deficiency) of 10, 22
Yellow Emperor's Canon of Medicine 1
Yin Qiao San (Powder of Lonicera and Forsythia) 46, 54
Yin 5, 9-10
   deficiency of 22
   exuberance of 5
Yin-yang 9-10
   balance of 16
   imbalance of 16
   interdependence of 9
   opposition of 9
   theory of 9-11
   transformation of 10
   waxing and waning of 10-11
Yu Ping Feng San (Jade-screen Powder) 30-31

Zhang Zhongjing 2
Zhen Jiu Jia Yi Jing (*A Classic of Acupuncture and Moxibustion*) 2

图书在版编目(CIP)数据

中医精萃:英文/谢竹藩著.
-北京:新世界出版社,1995.1
ISBN 7-80005-228-1

Ⅰ.中…
Ⅱ.谢…
Ⅲ.中医医学基础-英文
Ⅳ.R22

中 医 精 萃

谢竹藩 著

*

新世界出版社出版
(北京百万庄路24号)
北京大学印刷厂印刷
中国国际图书贸易总公司发行
(中国北京车公庄西路35号)
北京邮政信箱第399号 邮政编码100044
1995年(英文)第一版
ISBN 7-80005-228-1
02800
14-E-2923S